Civil society and health

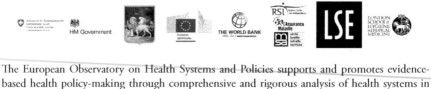

The European Observatory on Health Systems and Policies supports and promotes evidence-based health policy-making through comprehensive and rigorous analysis of health systems in Europe. It brings together a wide range of policy-makers, academics and practitioners to analyse trends in health reform, drawing on experience from across Europe to illuminate policy issues.

The European Observatory on Health Systems and Policies is a partnership between the WHO Regional Office for Europe; the Governments of Austria, Belgium, Finland, Ireland, Norway, Slovenia, Sweden, Switzerland, the United Kingdom and the Veneto Region of Italy; the European Commission; the World Bank; UNCAM (French National Union of Health Insurance Funds); the London School of Economics and Political Science; and the London School of Hygiene & Tropical Medicine.

Civil society and health

Contributions and potential

Edited by

Scott L. Greer
Matthias Wismar
Gabriele Pastorino
Monika Kosinska

European
Observatory
on Health Systems and Policies
a partnership hosted by WHO
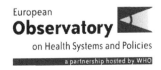

Keywords:
Public Health
Organizations
Cooperative Behavior
Community Participation

ISBN 978 92 890 5043 2

Printed in the United Kingdom

Cover design by M2M

Contents

List of figures, tables and boxes

Figures

Tables

Boxes

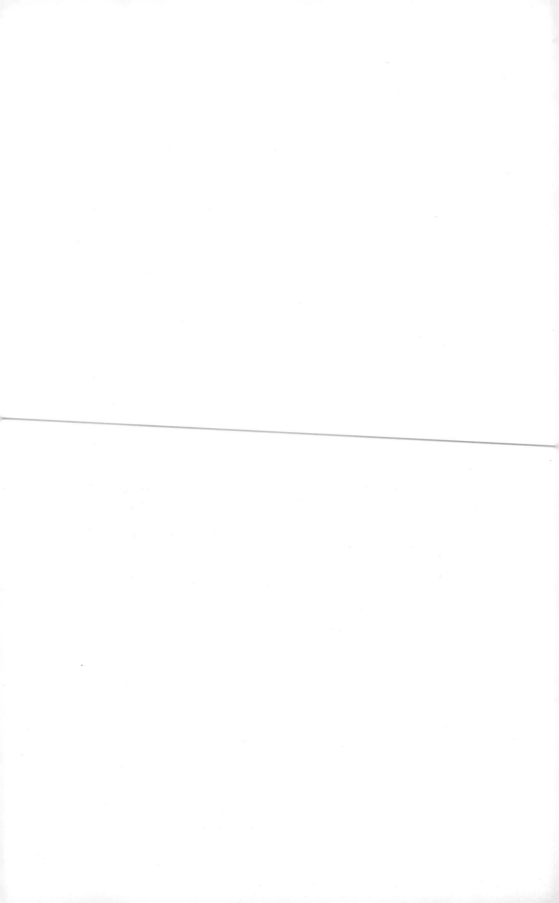

List of contributors

Maria Martin de Almagro is Marie Curie Postdoctoral Fellow at POLIS, University of Cambridge.

Natasha Azzopardi Muscat is Senior Lecturer at the Department of Health Services Management, University of Malta, Malta; and Consultant in Public Health Medicine at the Directorate for Health Information and Research, G'Mangia, Malta.

Erica Barbazza is Technical Officer at the WHO European Centre for Primary Health Care, Almaty, Kazakhstan.

Marleen Bekker is Senior Research Fellow in Governance and Innovation in Social Services (GAINS) at the Nijmegen School of Management, Radboud University, Nijmegen, the Netherlands.

Kirill Danishevskiy is Professor of the Higher School of Economics, Moscow, Russian Federation.

Michelle Falkenbach is a PhD Research Scholar of Health Management and Policy at the University of Michigan School of Public Health, Ann Arbor, USA.

Molly Green is a doctoral student at the University of Michigan School of Public Health, Ann Arbor, USA.

Scott L. Greer is Professor of Global Health Management and Policy at the University of Michigan School of Public Health, Ann Arbor, USA, and Senior Expert Adviser on Health Governance for the European Observatory on Health Systems and Policies, Brussels, Belgium.

Jan Kees Helderman is an Associate Professor of Governance and Innovation in Social Services (GAINS) at the Nijmegen School of Management, Radboud University, Nijmegen, the Netherlands.

Maria Jansen is Professor of Population Health at Maastricht University, Health Services Research Department, Maastricht, the Netherlands, and Programme Leader of the Academic Collaborative Centre for Public Health at the Public Health Service, South Limburg, Geleen, the Netherlands.

Maria Joachim is a PhD Research Scholar in Health Management and Policy at the University of Michigan, School of Public Health, Ann Arbor, USA.

Elizabeth J. King is Assistant Professor of Health Behaviour and Health Education at the University of Michigan School of Public Health and Associate Director of the Weiser Centre for Europe and Eurasia at the University of Michigan, Ann Arbor, USA.

Monika Kosinska is Programme Manager of Governance for Health at WHO Regional Office for Europe, Copenhagen, Denmark

Mark McCarthy is Emeritus Professor of Public Health Epidemiology & Public Health, University College London, United Kingdom.

Martin McKee is Professor of European Health at the London School of Hygiene and Tropical Medicine and Research Director of the European Observatory on Health Systems and Policies.

Natasa Maros is Project Coordinator at MyRight-Empowers people with disabilities, Sarajevo, Bosnia and Herzegovina.

Melita Murko is Technical Officer with the Mental Health Programme, WHO Regional Office for Europe, Copenhagen, Denmark.

Saime Ozcurumez is Associate Professor, Department of Political Science and Public Administration, Bilkent University, Ankara, Turkey.

Ilaria Passarani is Head of the Food and Health Department at the European Consumer Organization (BEUC), Brussels, Belgium, and Researcher at the Faculty of Health, Medicine and Life Sciences of Maastricht University, Maastricht, the Netherlands.

Gabriele Pastorino is Programme Management Officer, European Observatory on Health Systems and Policies, Brussels, Belgium.

Vesna-Kerstin Petrič is Head of Division for Health Promotion and Prevention of Non-communicable Diseases at the Ministry of Health, Ljubljana, Slovenia.

Maria D. Ramiro González is Medical Resident in Preventive Medicine and Public Health at the Hospital General Universitario Gregorio Marañón, Madrid, Spain.

Dirk Ruwaard is Professor of Public Health and Health Care Innovation and Chairman of the Department of Health Services Research as part of the Care and Public Health Research Institute (CAPHRI), Faculty of Health, Medicine and Life Sciences, Maastricht University, the Netherlands.

Andreas Schmid is Assistant Professor for Health Management at the University of Bayreuth, Germany.

Dinesh Sethi is Programme Manager for Violence and Injury Prevention at WHO Regional Office for Europe, Copenhagen, Denmark.

Kerry Waddell is Co-Lead Evidence Synthesis at the McMaster Health Forum, Hamilton, Canada

Matthias Wismar is Senior Health Policy Analyst at the European Observatory on Health Systems and Policies, Brussels, Belgium.

Deniz Yıldırım is a PhD Candidate in the Department of Political Science and Public Administration, Bilkent University, Ankara, Turkey.

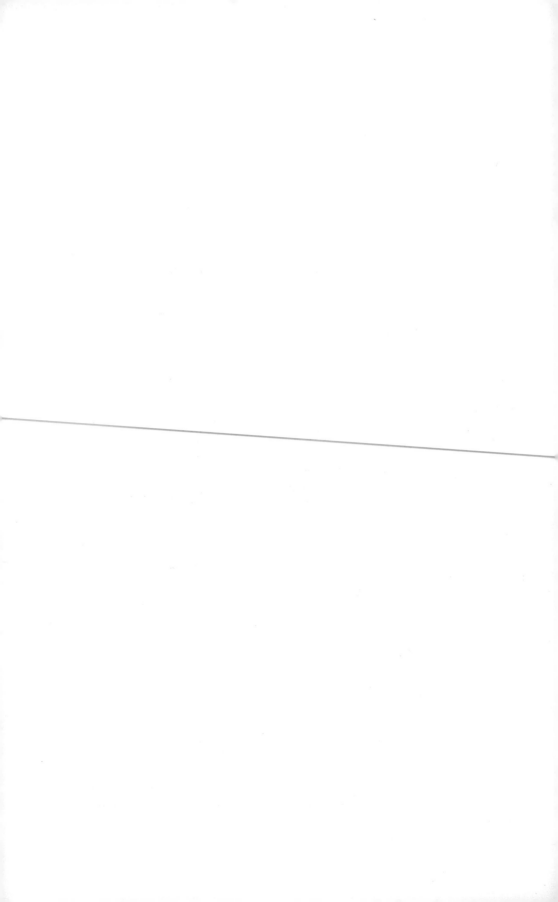

Acknowledgements

This volume has been commissioned and financially supported by the WHO Regional Office for Europe to assist the implementation of Health 2020, the regional health policy framework for Europe. We are grateful for all the support we received from Piroska Ostlin, divisional director for Policy and Governance for Health and Well-being, and her team.

We are grateful to all participants of the workshops we organized or attended to present and discuss conceptual frameworks and preliminary results.

We are very grateful to the Programme Managers of the WHO Regional Office for Europe who discussed with us our study in a workshop in December 2015 in Copenhagen. Some of them kept working with us on the study.

We would like to thank the participants of a workshop with European civil society organizations in April 2016 in Brussels, including Florence Berteletti, Sarada Das, Stella de Sabata, Pascal Garel, Andrea Glahn, Corinna Hartrampf, Willy J. Heuschen, Mervi Jokinen, Aagje Leven, Mathias Maucher, Mihaela Militaru, Patricia Munoz, Clive Needle, Dominick Nguyen, Ber Oomen, Robert Otok, Nina Renshaw, Mariann Skar, Jurate Svarcaite, Franz Terwey, Julia Wadoux, Jamie Wilkinson and Wendy Yared.

We are deeply indebted to Marleen Bekker, President of the Public Health Practice & Policy Section of EUPHA, the European Public Health Association. She included us in her workshop at the 2015 European Public Health Conference, Milan, Italy, and co-organized a pre-conference workshop on this publication at the EPH-Conference 2016 in Vienna. Her engagement has resulted in a sustained collaboration. Many thanks also to Kai Michelsen.

We drew inspiration from the international, intersectoral governance process initiated by WHO and supported by the French government. This included workshops and conferences in Paris in 2014, 2015 and 2016.

This volume has benefited substantially from our external reviewers Anne Hoel and Nina Renshaw. We are grateful for their thoroughness.

Many thanks to Adam Tiliouine, Annalisa Marianecci and all the many other colleagues at WHO and the Observatory for their technical and administrative support.

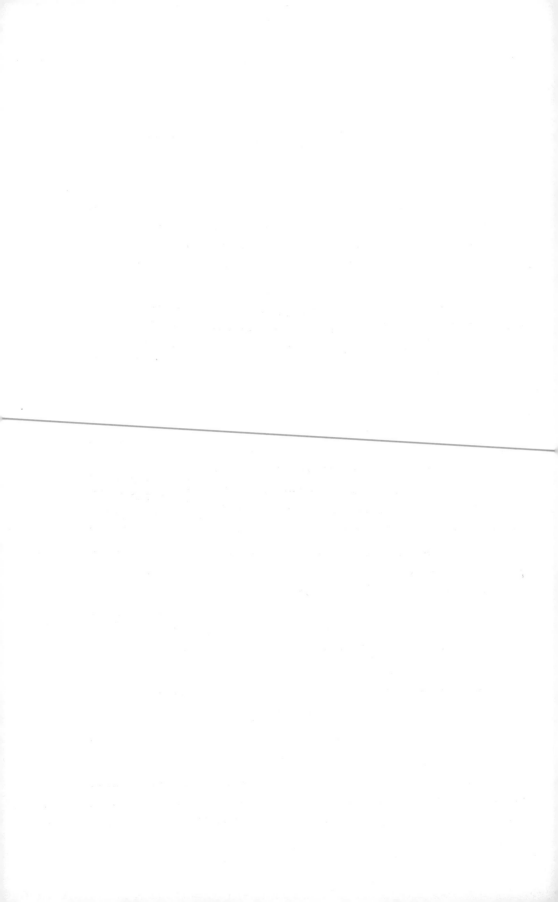

Foreword

One of the biggest challenges to meeting today's greatest health challenges is how to break the silos that dominate the planning, design, implementation, monitoring and evaluation of health strategies, programmes and activities. Too often these silos are dominated by a small group of experts in a top-down approach, without considering the wider stakeholders in the policy process or the equally important bottom-up approach. This means that it is the experts who identify the problems and formulate interventions, while the problems and solutions as perceived by those sectors who own the actions on important determinants of health, or those populations most affected rarely constitute the base for action.

Since its adoption in 2012, Health 2020, the European policy and strategy for health and well-being has inspired and supported action across countries in the European Region to strengthen the work across sectors to achieve health, well-being and health equity. Great strides are currently underway to increase the implementation of whole-of-government approaches, Health-in-all-policies and better governance for health and well-being. The next challenge for health policy makers is to strengthen the operationalization of the whole-of-society approach to health and well-being. In addition to key actors in for example local authorities, schools and employers, the role for civil society and representatives of target groups is essential to understand and support if we are to achieve our common goals and meet the challenges ahead.

We know that what needs to be changed is to have those targeted having the possibility to influence and control various determinants of health and to allow people to make their voices heard. Health policies and activities are most meaningful when target communities and groups are involved in all aspects of policy and programme development, implementation and evaluation. Creating resilient communities in which people are empowered and given the opportunity to express their needs and interests in the development of policy is one of the priority actions for the coming years and is at the heart of the successful achievement of the 2030 Agenda for Sustainable Development. In addition to this, civil society can respond quickly and with versatility to emerging health challenges and niche areas for health policy and play an essential role in acting as a bridge between the public sector and target communities.

This volume presents an essential overview to the plurality of civil society, its functions and contributions to health policy and service delivery, and showcases case studies that can help government authorities, institutions, organizations and individuals to build effective and sustainable partnerships with civil society.

Zsuzsanna Jakab
WHO Regional Director for Europe

Part I

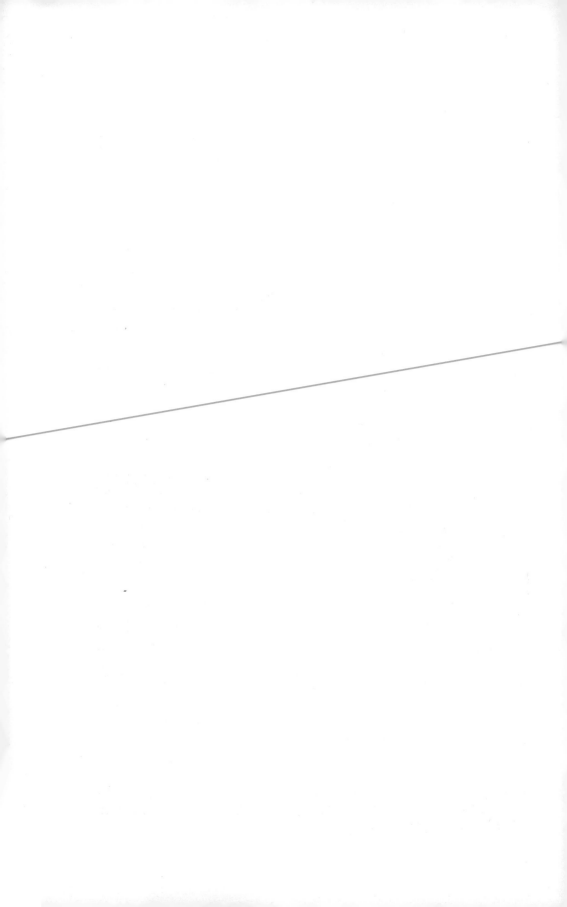

Chapter 1

What is civil society and what can it do for health?

Scott L. Greer, Matthias Wismar, Monika Kosinska

Fifty years ago "civil society" was a term known mostly to intellectual historians. Today, it has become a globally debated concept, the focus of a huge amount of argument and advocacy, and a part of politics and health in Europe whose importance is undisputed. Health policy-makers in Europe know that ignoring civil society has great perils and working with it has potential gains.

At global level and in some countries, working with civil society has become an established mechanism of health governance and governance for health. But many government-Civil Society Organization (CSO) collaborations are 'out of sync'. Representation does not fit, the governance of the relationship is often poor, the finance is inadequate, there are tensions between the public sector and the CSO, and administrative procedures are poorly harmonized (Buse & Harmer, 2007). Extolling civil society, or relying on it, is well and good, but creating a fruitful partnership presents a series of practical challenges.

Therefore, the basic question we are asking is, how can governments better work with civil society for health and health systems? To answer this question we also need to ask, what is the place of civil society in health? How can we address the practical challenges and advantages of working with CSOs across European societies? What are the contexts and instruments conducive and adequate to working with civil society? To address these questions we have developed concepts and analysis:

- a positive definition of CSOs;

- a matrix which helps to capture the diversity of civil society and its contribution and potential to policy-making, service delivery and governance of health and health systems;

- a set of seven case studies of CSOs in action tackling health and health system issues. The in-depth analysis focuses on the issues, the contributions, the instruments of engagements and the contexts; and

- a set of eight mini case studies to broaden the coverage of countries, types of civil society organization and issues tackled.

The authors are from academia and practical settings as well as WHO. In some cases they work in or with the aspect of civil society that they discuss. While this might be perceived as a conflict of interest, it is also an opportunity to tap their expertise and hear voices of civil society that would otherwise be excluded in a way that is not appropriate to a book about civil society's potential to contribute.

This chapter sets out in more detail the background to the study. It starts by explaining the concrete motivation of this book, which was inspired by Health 2020, the WHO European policy for health and well-being. The chapter provides a brief explanation of what civil society is, what it can do for health and health systems, and what particular benefits it may produce. The chapter also discusses the limits of civil society, and ends with a discussion of the principal instruments for engagement.

Chapter 2 presents the matrix, an analytical framework to map the territory of civil society and health. It also links different types of CSOs with different types of health and health system-related actions.

Chapter 3 brings together the definitions, conceptual frameworks and evidence presented throughout the volume. The chapter concludes that civil society is ubiquitous, diverse and beneficial. It then draws key lessons for regulating civil society and presents instruments for working with CSOs and suggests a practical framework for health policy-makers who wish to reach out and engage with civil society.

Chapter 4 to 10 present in-depth analysis of CSOs engaging for health and health systems. The chapters are complemented by mini case studies which are spread throughout the book. Together they showcase CSOs dealing with a large set of diverse issues such as tobacco control, access to pharmaceuticals in Europe and developing countries, the fall-out from austerity policies, the refugee crisis, HIV/AIDS, social partnerships, industry, corporal punishment, research policy, the hospice movement, obstetric care and stigma. The chapters and mini case studies come from Austria, Bosnia-Herzegovina, Belgium, Finland, Germany, Malta, the Netherlands, Poland, Russia, Slovenia, Turkey and the European Union.

1.1 Civil society, working with society and Health 2020

Working with society has become an important strategy for the WHO European Region. Health 2020, the new European policy for health and well-being for the 21st century, supported by several studies, is making the case for intersectoral, interdepartmental governance (McQueen et al., 2012; Kickbusch & Gleicher, 2012; WHO, 2012). Conceptually, this has been captured by the whole-of-government and the whole-of-society approach (Dubé et al., 2014).

When ministries of health are reaching out to other ministries and sectors in order to address the wider determinants of health outside their remit, they will need to build bridges between otherwise separated ministries and administration. They will need to establish dialogue and use intersectoral structures, such as public health ministers, parliamentary committees, cabinet committees, and interdepartmental committees for intersectoral actions (McQueen et al., 2012). But this whole-of government approach remains inside the government and administration and often does not reach civil society and the world of CSOs. To reach out to civil society and CSOs, the whole-of-society approach (WHO, 2012), which is at the centre of this scoping review, is needed.

Box 1.1 *The whole-of-society approach in Health 2020 (WHO, 2012)*

A whole-of-society approach goes beyond institutions; it influences and mobilizes local and global culture and media, rural and urban communities and all relevant policy sectors, such as the education system, the transport sector, the environment and even urban design, as demonstrated in the case of obesity and the global food system.

Whole-of-society approaches are a form of collaborative governance that can complement public policy. They emphasize coordination through normative values and trust-building among a wide variety of actors.

By engaging the private sector, civil society, communities and individuals, the whole-of-society approach can strengthen the resilience of communities to withstand threats to their health, security and well-being.

1.2 What is civil society?

Civil society is a concept with a long lineage in European social thought but it came into its own as a meaningful concept in politics in the 1980s (Gellner, 1994). That was the decade in which it gained recognition, and a very positive image, for a variety of reasons. It seemed to capture the promising nature of non-state organizations that were defying authoritarian regimes, especially in central and eastern Europe. It seemed also to form an alternative to the market-based world of the west, where the idea of non-commercial, volunteer activity offered political and policy options that were not thought to be available in market transactions. In both cases, the appeal of civil society was simple: it might allow politics and civil society to break out of simplistic frameworks, such as those of the state or the market and explore new possibilities.

Civil society therefore entered political conversation as a rather broad concept. It rapidly came to cover actors as diverse as trade unions in Communist Poland and Francoist Spain, the Lutheran Church in the German Democratic Republic and the participatory milieu of the 1980s left in the German Federal Republic. It was then expanded further as it went global, becoming both a key analytical tool for analysts of the decline of authoritarian regimes and a normative object of policy by governments and charities that sought to strengthen it worldwide. By the 1990s some had broadened it to include everything that was not formally part of the state, up to and including multinational corporations, while others had narrowed it down to a small set of designated organizations representing newer social movements born in the 1960s, and some others had narrowed it down still further into campaigning groups with little purchase on society. At the same time, efforts to promote civil society often fell afoul of its diversity. Trying to promote a confused and often very western concept (Gellner, 1994) in diverse societies as part of a broader mission of social change was a challenge for policy-makers and funders, and they did not always get what they wanted. The result was that civil society lost some of its popularity as a policy objective or a theoretical concept in the 21st century.

But the fact that civil society was a fad for policy-makers and professors alike does not mean that it is valueless. Far from it. It became such a popular concept because of its importance, variability and ubiquity in Europe.[1] It remains powerful – but it needs conceptual clarity, not another cycle of fashion.

Defining civil society is a large part of the problem of thinking about civil society.[2] We hoped to avoid many of the definitional disputes and normative arguments that bog down conversations about civil society. We started with a capacious definition, avoiding specific claims that are often too dependent on specific contexts or become tied up in philosophical issues removed from immediate policy concerns. As a result, we adopted an inclusive approach with weak exclusion criteria. We then divided civil society into rough categories of organizations and functions in order to highlight its diversity and contributions to different aspects of health, health care, and health policy. Not all kinds of organizations and not all kinds of functions are found in the civil

---

1 It is important to stress that we are writing for and about Europe. Civil society and arguments about civil society are highly context-dependent and hard to export. As a result, the experiences and meaning of civil society in other parts of the world remain outside our remit.

2 For a useful review of contemporary academic research and debates, see Anheier (2014) and Jensen (2006), and also the insightful first chapters of Kohler-Koch et al. (2013). For efforts to define and then measure civil society, see Heinrich (2005) and Malena & Volkhart (2007).

society of any given country. We also tried to avoid overly specific categories, since civil society organizations within any given country or political system tend to have distinctive legal and practical roles that do not translate more broadly. The point is to outline a framework that highlights the diversity and importance of civil society, point to different roles and relationships, and create a basic framework for discussing its role and contribution.

The core of a definition of civil society is that it is the society we engage in as active citizens, neither part of the market nor part of the state nor part of the family. "Neither state nor market" captures an essence of civil society, but it is hard to proceed without some more specific definitional characteristics. The next section explores that basic definition, which is the thread running through the many competitive definitions of civil society. It then refines the definition by identifying positive and contextual factors that mark civil society.

1.2.1 Neither state nor market nor family

The core of most sensible discussions of civil society – the point on which public intellectuals as different as Jürgen Habermas and Jeanne Kirkpatrick agree – is that it is part of neither the state nor the market (Habermas, 1975; Kirkpatrick, 1979).[3] It is obviously linked to both, for funding, legal status, and context, but it is also different, accountable neither to the state nor to the market.

Civil society is, like society, a blanket term for a much more concrete set of people and organizations. Civil society organizations (CSOs), rather than civil society, are the real locus of civil society and where it happens. To characterize the civil society of a country is to characterize its CSOs and their interactions with each other and broader society. To work with civil society is to work with CSOs. To complain of civil society, or try to change it, is to challenge, join, or create CSOs.

Civil society: definition

Civil society is seen as a social sphere separate from both the state and the market. The increasingly accepted understanding of the term civil society organizations (CSOs) is that of non-state, not-for-profit, voluntary organizations formed by people in that social sphere.

---

3 The origins of the concept focused much more on distinguishing it from family as a form of social organization, though some thinkers still consider family to be part of civil society. This distinction mattered less in Europe of the 1780s than it does now, and we accordingly give it somewhat less emphasis in this particular discussion. That is not to downplay its theoretical importance or its potential importance when discussing social organization outside Europe (or even to discourage inquiry into the place of families in European societies). For influential intellectual histories with less immediate practical relevance, see Cohen & Arato (1994) and Keane (2013).

Being "neither state nor market" is an enormously diverse category – even more diverse than categories such as "business". That is one reason for the rise and fall of the concept of civil society, and the difficulty of defining it. This definition encompasses the most corporatist of social partners, such as the unions and trades associations that govern so much of life in Austria, to the most specific advocacy groups for vulnerable populations such as the homeless. As a result, the real challenge is not to theorize the abstract relationship between civil society, the market, and the state. There is not much we can usefully say about the problems and potential of Austrian trade unions, Cypriot "social groceries" for the hungry, and Royal Colleges in the UK in the abstract. But then, there is not much we can abstractly say about the public administrations or economies of Austria, Cyprus, and the UK. The real challenge is to understand the civil society of a given place, its relationship to health, and its potential to further improve health. And that will require specificity, context, and a willingness to examine cases in detail. The rest of this chapter will identify issues that do fit with civil society in the abstract, but also highlight the diversity of its nature and its roles in society.

Examples of civil society organizations

Activist groups, charities, civic groups, campaigns, sports clubs, social clubs, community foundations, community/local associations, consumer organizations, cooperatives, churches, cultural groups, environmental groups, foundations, lobbies, men's groups, policy institutions, political parties, private voluntary organizations, professional associations, religious organizations, social associations, social enterprises, support groups, trade unions, voluntary associations, women's groups.

1.2.2 Positive characteristics

"Neither state nor market nor family" encompasses much of human life, from chess players in the park to organized religion. How can we go beyond that to start identifying civil society organizations so that we know what we are discussing and how it fits in with policy?

We will start with positive characteristics to complement the negative definition of 'neither state nor market'. It is worth noting again that the contexts and forms of civil society are so diverse as to make it hard to produce a useful definition that spans all the world's societies, so we are here focusing on the situation in the European region. That allows us to specify with more precision what does and does not constitute a manifestation of civil society.

We start with *autonomy*: the extent to which the organization determines what it is for and whom it serves. Autonomy distinguishes a CSO from profit-making companies (e.g. public affairs consultancies) or arms of the government.[4] Key questions that we may ask of organizations in order to determine whether they have the autonomy to be called CSOs include:

- *Who has the power to shut down the organization?*
  A CSO is not autonomous if somebody else can close it down.

- *Who has the power to choose and dismiss its leader (e.g. chief executive)?*
  A CSO is not autonomous if it cannot select and reject its leadership.

- *Who has the power to stipulate its statutes and operating by-laws?*
  A CSO is not autonomous if it cannot stipulate its own internal procedures, including issues such as determination of budget and priorities.

- *What is its economic base?*
  Ideally, members. It is quite possible to depend on philanthropists, governments, or others for resources, but insofar as an organization depends on them, it should expect as a matter of realism to have its autonomy questioned and should have a compelling answer to those questions, typically involving transparency and separation between funders and decision-making.

- *Who has the power to determine its mandate?*
  Finally, autonomy requires that an organization must not have its mandate determined for it, or that an externally defined mandate may be something at its foundation that it outgrows.

In some legal systems, organizations must make their answers clear and there are legal and regulatory mechanisms to constrain the nature of such organizations. Formality does not always make the real answers clear, but it is a place to start in determining whether an organization is a CSO or something else. If nothing else, identifying discrepancies between formal and real behaviour is a useful way to understand what really runs an organization. Likewise, informal CSOs exist and often do important work. Even if there is no equivalent to a formal mandate or set of bylaws, or even if the formal documentation is unenlightening, it is possible to ask for the informal equivalent – to ask what the organization is for, who leads it and why it does what it does. A definition that fits all the different organizations, contexts, societies and questions would be impossibly unwieldy, but these questions sketch the limits of what an organization can do, and direct our attention to the contextual factors of civil society.

---

4 Known in some circles as GONGOs: Government-organized non-governmental organizations. It is telling that Trägårdh and Witoszek can supply a whole lexicon of such sarcastic acronyms, including DONGO (donor-organized NGO), BONGO (business-organized NGO), PONGO (party-organized NGO), etc. Lots of people, it seems, would like to tap the credibility, funding streams and organizational forms of civil society.

Balancing autonomy against other desirables – such as funding, political engagement, credibility, and the institutionalization necessary to deliver complex projects and employ staff – is always a challenge.

The second positive characteristic, after autonomy, is the link to a *constituency*. This can be a *representative* link, in which the organization engages in policy debates on behalf of that organization, or it can be a link to a *community* that it services with some kind of benefit or function. Many organizations are both in some measure: they both represent and provide services to the community. In less formal cases, it is often hard to distinguish the two activities. But organizations that neither represent nor provide services to an identifiable community are suspect.

In short, civil society is made up of organizations *that are autonomous, that are not wholly of the state, market, or family, and that work with or for a given constituency that can be identified*. Further elaboration of this definition, such as tighter exclusion or inclusion criteria, should be context-dependent since what works in one place might not work in another.

Civil society has to be defined in the context of government, market, and family. This naturally limits the specificity of a definition, since civil society's roles, access to politics, ability to influence society, independence from commercial interests, and strength are all context-dependent. There is a European Union civil society because there is a European Union political system that can define and be influenced by civil society, and there is a French or Lithuanian civil society because there are French and Lithuanian states and societies that can define civil society and in which civil society can play a role. The importance of context means, though, that autonomy and constituency operate differently. Being neither state nor market nor family ultimately means that the shape of civil society depends on the nature of state, market, and family.

Apart from academic discussion, the important consequences of definitions of civil society and non-governmental organization can be demonstrated by the WHO framework of engagement with non-state actors (FENSA) (see Box 1.2.). FENSA defines NGOs and other non-state actors in order to clarify on the principles, benefits and risks of engagement. It also defines to what extent WHO can interact with the different non-state actors regarding participation, evidence, advocacy and technical collaboration.

1.3 What does civil society do for health?

The fundamental case for the role of civil society in health in Europe is that it is *ubiquitous, diverse, and beneficial*. States, markets and families do not

---

Box 1.2 *Non-governmental organizations and other non-state actors according to the WHO framework of engagement with non-state actors (FENSA)*

8. For the purpose of this framework, non-State actors are nongovernmental organizations, private sector entities, philanthropic foundations and academic institutions.

9. **Nongovernmental organizations** are non-profit entities that operate independently of governments. They are usually membership-based, with non-profit entities or individuals as members exercising voting rights in relation to the policies of the nongovernmental organization, or are otherwise constituted with non-profit, public-interest goals. They are free from concerns which are primarily of a private, commercial or profit-making nature. They could include, for example, grassroots community organizations, civil society groups and networks, faith-based organizations, professional groups, disease-specific groups, and patient groups.

10. **Private sector entities** are commercial enterprises, that is to say businesses that are intended to make a profit for their owners. The term also refers to entities that represent, or are governed or controlled by, private sector entities. This group includes (but is not limited to) business associations representing commercial enterprises, entities not "at arm's length" from their commercial sponsors, and partially or fully State-owned commercial enterprises acting like private sector entities.

International business associations are private sector entities that do not intend to make a profit for themselves but represent the interests of their members, which are commercial enterprises and/or national or other business associations. For the purposes of this framework, they shall have the authority to speak for their members through their authorized representatives. Their members shall exercise voting rights in relation to the policies of the international business association.

11. **Philanthropic foundations** are non-profit entities whose assets are provided by donors and whose income is spent on socially useful purposes. They shall be clearly independent from any private sector entity in their governance and decision-making.

12. **Academic institutions** are entities engaged in the pursuit and dissemination of knowledge through research, education and training.

Source: http://www.who.int/about/collaborations/non-state-actors/A69_R10-FENSA-en.pdf?ua=1, accessed 12 June 2017.

---

do all the work that contributes to health, or might not do it especially well. States are financially constrained and good public administration will often, by design, emphasize equality, accountability, and deliberation over speed and experimentation. Markets, ultimately, demand that something be profitable if it is to attract resources. Families look after their own better than others.

Much that contributes to health is therefore best done by neither state nor market nor family. Emblematically, neither advocacy nor services to rapidly changing distinct vulnerable populations are ways to make money or show public administrations at their best, and vulnerable populations frequently cannot rely on families. Nobody questions the ability of the French or German state to provide services to migrants, but civil society organizations could start to provide services much more quickly than the state when the Syrian refugee crisis began (see mini case study 6 after Chapter 9).

Even when the best eventual solution is the market or the state, the way to the solution is often shown by civil society organizations with their ability to experiment and focus on the job, rather than being constrained by the demands of formal politics or profit. The ancestors of most western health systems, for example, are to be found in various forms of civil society association that started to provide health benefits.

Chapter 2 discusses the diverse contributions of civil society to health and health policy. For health, civil society can deliver services that governments are unwilling or unable to deliver because of lack of political interest, inflexible public administrations, resource constraints or lack of trust in certain populations. It can often offer committed people, flexibility, and responsiveness in service delivery that public sector and private sector organizations alike fail to muster. It can also mediate problematic policies, whether through a role in implementation or through assisting populations in dealing with a problem. With its low cost of entry, it can also be innovative and responsive, with civil society organizations addressing new tasks quickly and sometimes developing the solutions that will eventually be adopted by bigger public and private organizations. Civil society can therefore compensate for policy failures, through quick responses and incubation of alternative organizational models. Finally, civil society organizations often play a key role in advocacy, trying to drive social change through direct campaigns on topics such as disease awareness or public health issues such as smoking and domestic violence (Chao, 2005).

For health policy, meanwhile, civil society can bring expertise, ideas, and diverse perspectives. It is unfair to ask civil society organizations to "represent" groups as if civil society were a parliament, but it is wholly legitimate to appreciate the expertise and views they bring, especially when they come from smaller segments of society that might not be heard in an electoral process or party politics. That is why a policy that has the approval of, or at least has been discussed with, relevant civil society organizations is often seen to be more credible. The most immediately affected interests have been asked for their views and information, which in general means the policy will be better thought-through, targeted, and perhaps implemented (Putnam, 1993). A policy that is pushed through in the face of opposition from affected civil society groups might be perfectly legitimate, but it will also be contentious and face difficulties.

It is undeniable that most governments find some aspects of civil society more attractive than others. Low-cost delivery is attractive to policy-makers with constrained budgets, but advocacy, new ideas, and efforts to shape the political agenda are all uncomfortable and can be regarded as beside the point if the government has already decided what it wants to do. Connection with less powerful and more vulnerable groups in society can lead to broad benefits but it can also empower them in ways that incumbent powers find uncomfortable. Consulting civil society organizations can provide some information, even if it is only information about opposition to the policy. Still, the reason to engage with civil society is that it might make health policy better and it is probably impossible to have the benefits of civil society without being critiqued by some of its members. If governments want civil servants, they can hire civil servants, but if they work with civil society, as they almost inevitably will, they must cope with criticism and an element of unpredictability that comes with commitment and flexibility.

The comfort and discomfort of working with civil society also varies by context. For example, in much of central and western Europe there is a long tradition of social partnership in which unions, employer associations, and the state are jointly involved in governing the economy (Chapter 9). Unions and employer associations in this context are civil society organizations that play a key role in making the government function, and their activity as repeat players in governance can feel quite different from smaller advocacy groups or international CSOs protesting policy from the outside. The relations between government and civil society are endlessly variable and can always be made more cooperative, more argumentative, more transparent or more trusting. The burden of doing so is often more on policy-makers than on civil society, for it is often the behaviour of policy-makers and governments that has undermined trust and perhaps even created the gaps that civil society fills. Nonetheless, better partnership is possible.

1.4 Benefits of civil society engagement

What are some of the benefits of civil society engagement that relationships should respect and enhance – or could impair? There are a few overarching themes: empowerment, service delivery, commitment, flexibility, participation in policy, and credibility.

Empowerment is a key benefit of a strong civil society both in general and in the health context. The Marmot Review defined empowerment as material, psycho-social, and political, the latter not necessarily or primarily meaning formal engagement in politics (Marmot & Bell, 2012; Marmot et al., 2010). Empowerment is strongly correlated with health and well-being, and its absence, whether due to poverty, illness, or stressful working conditions, is a cause of ill health, as Marmot has demonstrated (Marmot, 2004). Many conditions of modern life are in some way disempowering, and addressing disempowerment is important both to health and to a successful, sustainable, thriving society. It is here that civil society comes in.

In terms of social benefits, empowerment through civil society creates opportunities for people of many different kinds to empower themselves by acting together (a theme of many of the mini case studies in this book, which range from disability rights campaigns in Bosnia to Polish mothers seeking better obstetrical care). Effective participation in formal politics and policy in particular tends to be an expensive, specialist activity. Effective participation in civil society, and participation in politics through civil society, is often much easier and more attractive because of the diversity and entrepreneurialism of civil society organizations. Knowing about and participating in a consultation on local health services, for example, requires energy, optimism, and specialist skills that an individual citizen will often lack, but a group of citizens can jointly develop. The result is that a strong civil society, *by empowering citizens*, is a component of a strong democracy – a point first noted by de Tocqueville and scarcely put better since (de Tocqueville & Goldhammer, 2004).

Engagement with a strong civil society can also have specific benefits in the context of a health care system. Being a patient or having a chronic condition can often be a disempowering experience in all sorts of ways (Parsons, 1975; Pilnick & Dingwall, 2011), from financial costs to social isolation and physical pain. Patients and carers who organize to share information can reduce these burdens and empower themselves, whether to manage their disease better or to improve the quality and access of their care. If the health care system often deals with disempowered people and disempowers them still more, then patient, carer, and community groups in civil society can help to reverse that disempowerment.

Service delivery is perhaps the most common attraction for policy-makers. Civil society delivers things that state, market, and family cannot deliver – from well-run health care facilities to credible ethical determinations to outreach to vulnerable populations, social campaigns, and volunteers. Delivery, doing what others cannot, is a key part of the relationship between health systems and civil society almost everywhere (see, for example, Chapters 6 and 7 on how civil society responded to austerity in Cyprus and the refugee crisis in Turkey). This means that there are key kinds of relationships to be managed, with consequences of all sorts. First of all, how is a partnership to work? Is it to be in the form of grants or contracts? Who will determine the goals? How much oversight will the public sector expect, and how much should there be? What are the drawbacks for a CSO of becoming a contractor? Secondly, there are others who want delivery from CSOs, such as international donors and organizations. The same questions exist for them, but everybody involved in such a relationship must also balance multiple political arenas from local to global to the politics of donors in entirely different countries (whose interest in a given problem or country might be fleeting or based on some misapprehensions). Thirdly, the more a CSO is delivering according to government or other funder priorities, the more it risks its autonomy, which in turn might risk other virtues such as commitment, knowledge, and credibility.

Commitment. Part of the reason civil society organizations can (and often do) work so well is a factor that state and market cannot tap: the commitment of people who are called to a mission, people who are working for a group or cause that they believe in. Commitment is part of the reason civil society organizations do things that state, market, and family will never do, and it is part of the reason why their autonomy is so important. Commitment demands that the organization is doing something that its donors and volunteers believe in, since otherwise they might demand market wages or public sector benefits. In other words, one of the most dangerous phases for a CSO is when its activities become so large-scale, so important to others, or so bureaucratized that its volunteers lose the sense that it belongs to them. Such an organization risks losing much of what makes it special.

Flexibility. The cost of entry to civil society is very low in most cases. If there is no special barrier put in the way, it is easy for a few people to form a local group and clean up a park or advocate that it have better playground equipment. This low cost of entry, which is further lowered in societies where there is high trust and extensive civil society engagement already (Putnam, 1993; Goldberg, 1996), means that it is often civil society that responds first to a crisis, as in the mini case study of refugee accommodation in this book (mini case study 6, after Chapter 9), or that responds to unexpected new needs, as in the austerity case study in this book (see Chapter 6). As the case study of austerity in Cyprus suggests, civil society organizations that are already entrenched in delivery and contracts with government might be more flexible than the public sector but they are still often less flexible than more spontaneous and less institutionalized organizations.

Participation in policy. One of the key benefits of a strong civil society is that it can bring new *information* to decision-makers, whether through research, through close contacts with particular populations, or through bringing opinions that are born neither in the state nor in the private sector. The benefits to policy-makers of civil society participation in policy-making are not just better information and better legitimacy, however. The benefits also include *diverse ideas* that their employees might not originate.

The ability of CSOs to bring any kind of information and ideas into policy-making, however, depends on the existence of mechanisms suited to their resources (see Chapter 5 on the European Medicines Agency's engagement strategies, and mini case studies 3 and 4). There is an almost infinite variety of consultation mechanisms to involve civil society, including consultative forums and publication of government proposals for comment, and less formal mechanisms such as listening tours by officials. These need not be broad consultative forums. Sometimes the most effective participation is in narrow forums where civil society organizations can exchange ideas with policy-makers on specific topics such as food regulation, homelessness, or professional regulation (recalling that groups wholly composed of and accountable to business, with no broader accountability for social outcomes, are not part of civil society even when they share similar organizational features). Likewise, participation mechanisms make sense only in the context of the broader political system; the narrow forums for technical conversation in France make sense in that country's policy-making just as the broad consultation documents of the European Union make sense in EU policy-making (Page, 2012). In particular, there is a distinction between civil society as a source of *representatives*, who can speak for a particular community, and *experts*, who can contribute a less or differently biased view.

Credibility. In political theory, a government has all the legitimacy it needs from its election, but in practice, many policies are challenged if they were made without the participation of affected interests, which are often best accessed through their organization in civil society (Greer, Wismar & Figueras, 2016). As a result, civil society's credibility matters, and that comes from its participation and endorsement. Politicians are good at politics, by definition. They know how to empower interests to work after they move on. They also, therefore, know how to harness CSOs to make them do things and borrow the legitimacy of civil society. Creating opportunities for civil society to hold governments to account for their commitment is a basic technique used by ministers who want their innovations to persist after they move on (Greer & Lillvis, 2014).

In summary, the engagement of civil society with health policy and health is substantially dependent on the legal and political framework, which can affect both the benefits that civil society can bring and the ability of the political system and health system to hear and benefit from them. Civil society is often committed, diverse, and bottom-up, but the political, legal, and institutional context in both government and health system can lead to great variation in how it engages and whether the benefits of civil society engagement are realized.

1.5 The limits of civil society engagement

CSOs are heterogeneous and so are the interests they represent. They may have conflicting ideas about policy development and agenda building; they may deal differently with systematic and anecdotal evidence; and some of them are just not compatible with mandated government policy. For example, with regards to vaccination CSOs have played ambiguous roles, some even sowing confusion and doubts, for example on measles or on HIVP (Laurent-Ledru, Thomson & Monsonego, 2011). Some organizations representing citizens and patients have been criticized for opacity regarding their funding sources and lines of accountability, raising suspicions that vested interests are using CSOs as a vehicle to undermine certain policies, such as tobacco control policies, or to push certain medicinal products into the market place. The uses and abuses of civil society will be dealt with as a cross-cutting theme throughout the chapters of this volume.

While most countries agree that participation and democracy have a value as such, and must be supported in all sectors and contexts, there is much less consensus on depth and breadth of public involvement. Some countries have implemented referendum procedures to ensure that citizens' organizations can voice discontent and compel policy-makers to deal with the issues. There are plenty of other ways of informing, hearing or allowing citizens' participation in policy development. Examples include citizens' representatives' participation in health services commissioning and decommissioning decisions, and formalized mediation procedures in environmental impact assessments. Some commentators have argued that civil society participation is a key strategy to revive western democracies (Crouch et al., 2001). Others have argued that participation is a key strategy to create ownership and ensure legitimacy of otherwise contentious decisions in highly diversified societies. But there are also doubts and dilemmas about the legitimacy of CSO influence.

A credible civil society comes from its autonomy from the state and market, even if it can gain from the endorsement and attention of government and the resources of businesses. Governments can influence civil society, through contracting relationships, legal regulation, and participatory mechanisms. But it is worth remembering that the benefits of civil society engagement come partly from its independence from the state. *A credible civil society is necessary if its endorsement is to make policy more credible.* If it is replaying policy-makers' own messages, it will not be bringing new ideas; nor will it necessarily be credible as a messenger. Civil society organizations have to compete with others in society, above or below ground, to represent different voices. Once shielded from competition, they will often cease to represent anybody and will have little to contribute to policy debates. That means policy-makers should be attentive – if civil society organizations are saying inconvenient things, it might be for a good reason. By the same token, civil society organizations can often be infiltrated by private commercial interests. A legal framework that provides some clarity about their origins and membership will generally help to make such interests transparent.

Finally, there is little general reason to think that civil society is a panacea. The equivalence between a strong civil society and harmonious democracy, popularized by Putnam (Putnam, 1993), is facile. As Mann noted, German civil society in the 1930s was, "led by Nazis, a strong but evil civil society . . . Civil society may not be very civil!" (Mann, 2004; Satyanath, Voigtlaender & Voth, 2013). Put another way, "'civil society' and 'uncivil society' cannot be separated" (Pedahzur & Weinberg, 2001).

There are two key points to be made here. First, civil society can strengthen or undermine democracy and intergroup relations. A fruitful way to think about the difference is that civil society can bridge social cleavages (for example, by bringing together members of different religious groups in a shared sporting league) or can reinforce them (by, for example, having separate sporting leagues for each religious community)(Varshney, 2001). The latter is pernicious and endangers the stability of the political system, while the former lessens the risk of instability and ethnic conflict. Secondly, Putnam's influential work, which found that the quality of government within Italy varied with the strength of civil society, was somewhat mistitled. The book was called *Making Democracy Work*, but on the evidence in it, which was largely about public administration, a better title would have been *Making Public Administration* Work (Putnam, 1993; Goldberg, 1996). For the purposes of this book, the fact that civil society contributes to better and more responsive public services, which Putnam's book largely demonstrates, is the most important factor.

1.6 How does civil society engage with health?

No organization exists in a vacuum, and civil society occupies a vast space around the power centres of politics and the economy. That is why it is so hard to define; it is not just as protean as human life, it is also able to grow in very different social, political, and economic contexts.

The positive and contextual aspects of civil society that we listed earlier started to identify the mechanisms that connect civil society, health systems, health policy and health. Any sensible analysis of civil society in health must contend with all of these contextual factors, asking for each one what it does to give civil society its shape. In them often lies the key to a more productive relationship. Any sensible effort to work with civil society organizations involves understanding both their context and their positive characteristics. The context might not always enable all the positive characteristics that partners could want.

How is civil society connected to broad health and health policies? How, in other words, can policy-makers best work with civil society? This is one of the most important questions for civil society, for there are many different types of possible relationships, and they range from friendly to oppositional and positive to dysfunctional. We start here with the contextual factors:

Freedom of association. The underlying right that makes civil society possible is the right to associate in groups. This right is therefore often targeted by regimes seeking less democratic input and a less empowered citizenry (for example, Franco's Spain required a permit for any non-religious gathering of more than twenty people, even including family events, which pushed civil society into the Catholic Church (Greer, 2016)).

Regulatory and legal issues shape the kinds of CSOs that exist, what they can do, and how flexible their relationships can be. What is the basic legal status of civil society organizations? How many different legal statuses are available to them and what are the implications? Are there policies designed to aid civil society activity, such as tax exemptions? Legal questions are often overlooked in high-level discussions of civil society, but they matter. They influence the ease of starting a CSO, the long-term governance and organizational stability of CSOs, the financial resources of CSOs, the advocacy and participation implications of CSOs, the scale of CSO dependence on smaller donors and members versus public, wealthy, or international funders, and the ability of CSOs to formulate and change their missions. It is worth distinguishing between *legal* – involving legislation, the legal profession, and the courts – and *regulatory* – involving government and regulatory instruments – because they often have different dynamics and pressure points. In general, trying to set a broad legal framework and letting diversity work is better than trying to micro-engineer civil society organizations and their work. Micro-engineering endangers much of what civil society brings in the first place, which includes diversity and responsiveness to diverse groups and people.

As a result, the first step is making the case for an *effective, formal, transparent and efficient system for registering civil society organizations*. Effective, meaning that it is responsive and has enough coverage and benefits to attract CSOs and reflect them; formal, meaning that it is based in law, can be understood by an intelligent outsider, and is not subject to private manipulation; transparent, meaning that decisions and their grounds are made clear; and efficient, meaning that it does not demand much resourcing or distort civil society activities. There are many such systems in operation, whether under specific charity laws, or company registration laws, or tax laws. Such a system can also allow them to gain benefits, such as tax benefits or access to youths doing civilian service. While making registration transparent, formal and efficient decreases the costs of registration, it is not useful to demand that every organization in civil society must register, since many of them go through what we might regard as a trial stage of informal organization, and not everybody wants to enter into formal contact with the state no matter what the benefits may be.

Once there is a system of some sort, we can then ask that it effectively ensures the autonomy of civil society. For example, we can ask that CSOs file bylaws, financial accounts, and a constitution, and even allow them to be challenged if they fail to abide by those rules. Even if an organization clearly "works for" somebody, at least the formal system can make that clearer.

Financing in its various forms is important. Civil society organizations are funded by a wide variety of mechanisms, including small donations, large donors, international organizations, their own endowments, membership fees, sales of products and services, contracts for service provision with the state or private actors, and grants for projects. CSOs can be adept at obtaining resources in kind, such as volunteer work, and likewise can have an impact at prices that private and public sector actors would find impossible, but ultimately much of civil society needs money, and areas like health care provision need a lot of it.

The problems of financing civil society are endless and, again, context-dependent. Maintaining intellectual and practical autonomy from rich donors, government contracts, and other revenue measures can be hard. Competition for funds can keep civil society streamlined, relevant, and evolving, but core funding can enable long-term investments and reduce dependence on donors' fads. Likewise, accountability can be difficult to ensure for organizations that enjoy their own resource base (such as an endowment) or lucrative economic franchises (such as insurance sales or lotteries). The source of revenue can bias the effectiveness, views, and broad credibility of a CSO, but is also very difficult to ensure on a top-down basis. There will always be many CSOs who frustrate somebody with their dependence, and others that frustrate with their independence.

There are two kinds of problems in particular. One is the relationship of civil society with businesses. By definition, civil society organizations are not state actors, and people motivated by a cause will often have a different kind of credibility from businesses. As a result, it is a simple and often rewarding strategy for business interests to portray themselves as civil society – what Americans sometimes call "Astroturfing" (Astroturf is a brand name for artificial grass); in other words, creating an artificial grassroots base. Transparency about funding is an important part of establishing autonomy from the market. Long-term credibility is more important still. Funding sources can always be questioned, which is why a record of independence and clear accountability often matters more to the reputation and importance of a group. Strong civil societies will often police themselves, by extending or denying credibility to other organizations. Over time, it generally becomes quite clear what is grass and what is Astroturf.

Secondly, there is the relationship between civil society and the state. Here, there are a number of problems. In particular, the state often has a great deal of power over civil society. Not only does it set and enforce the basic legal framework for civil society, it also sets the terms of political participation and often finances civil society organizations. The result is a constant stream of efforts by those with independent sources of finance (businesses, wealthy donors) or by the government itself to use contracts and grants to civil society organizations as ways to influence their work. Governments might give contracts to civil society organizations like universities because they want their commitment, knowledge, and credibility, but then find themselves funding their own critics. It is all too tempting to value the short-term and try to constrain civil society, with ill effects on policy decisions and the ability of civil society to deliver anything people or the state might ask of it.

Political contexts fall into two basic categories: what does the government want civil society to do and how well can it enforce its wishes; and how does civil society fit into the broader way of policy-making in a given country? The first question is a big one. Here it is worth noting that civil society of some description exists almost everywhere, and does something useful even if governments do not appreciate it. The second question, concerning how well civil society fits into policy development, is a question about politicization and the autonomy of civil society from political action. It is easy for CSOs to enter into what are basically clientelistic political relations, working for parties or individual politicians as conduits for money or support. Some societies that are organized by political party families have worked extremely well (for example, in postwar Austria), but it is not the norm. The problem is akin to the problem of politicizing the civil service and filling its posts with patronage appointees – there can be short-term benefits, but in the long run the risk is that neither the public service nor civil society will function well if they work for party politicians.

In particular, the closeness of the connection between civil society and the state involves a number of trade-offs and it is hard to say when the right trade-off has been made. On one hand, civil society organizations gain credibility when they are interlocutors of the state, but on the other hand they gain credibility from autonomy vis-à-vis the state. Civil society can be instrumentalized by political and partisan actors, but over time that endangers the commitment, flexibility, and low cost that make CSOs a desirable way to deliver services. It can be turned into an echo chamber for the government, or even shut down, but that diminishes the flow of ideas in society, makes government more fragile and error-prone, reduces the resilience of society by disempowering people and reducing the diversity of ideas, and leaves government less capable of engaging with or answering the range of needs and people in society.

Social contexts are multifarious, but in the context of relating to civil society there is one key point worth emphasizing: civil society can fill in important gaps, will frequently do so unbidden and can be a key partner if supported. For example, we can imagine a society in which some combination of strong family structures and a welfare state mean that most citizens enjoy appropriate access to health care. But what about the ones who are not fully integrated into the labour market, who are estranged from their families, or who suffer discrimination? Civil society organizations can represent them and work for them in ways that the surrounding society and political structures cannot or will not.

1.7 Summing up the background to the study on civil society and health

This book sets out to map the place of civil society in health. It uses a set of case studies and a broad framework to make three key points. First, it highlights the *ubiquity and diversity of civil society*. Civil society means many things, many kinds of organizations and many kinds of tasks. It does not mean the same thing in any two political systems, and so what it contributes and can contribute also varies. Secondly, it highlights the *importance of context in understanding civil society's diversity and contributions*. What does civil society do in a given place, what has it traditionally done, what could it do, and why? These are all empirical questions. They also mean that it can be unwise to try to export a form or function of civil society from one country to another. Everybody likes to export their own institutions and ideas, but those institutions and ideas might be actively harmful, or at least have significant opportunity costs, in other settings. Thirdly, it highlights the *broad value of civil society* in many aspects of life, from social resilience to informed policy-making and good quality technical standard setting. Few countries are without civil society, and there are benefits to health in working with it.

In the subsequent chapters and mini case studies throughout the book, we highlight concrete cases of civil society at work, showing the diversity of civil society and its tasks, its broad value, and the importance of understanding context in understanding its work and potential. We do not aspire to cover every cell in the matrix from this chapter, and nor does Chapter 2 aspire to cover every kind of civil society action. Rather, the purpose is to show the ubiquity, diversity, and beneficial aspects of civil society in different health policy contexts.

References

Anheier HK (2014). Civil Society Research: Ten Years on. *Journal of Civil Society*, 10(4):335–339. doi: 10.1080/17448689.2014.984973.

Buse K, Harmer AM (2007). Seven habits of highly effective global public–private health partnerships: practice and potential. *Social science & medicine*, 64(2):259–271.

Chao E (2005). A study in social change: The Domestic Violence Prevention Movement in Taiwan. *Critical Asian Studies*, 37(1):29–50. doi: 10.1080/1467271052000305250.

Cohen JL, Arato A (1994). *Civil Society and Political Theory*. Cambridge, MA, MIT Press.

de Tocqueville A, Goldhammer A (2004). *Democracy in America*. New York, Library of America.

Crouch C et al. (2001). Conclusions: the future of citizenship. In: Crouch C et al. eds. *Citizenship, Markets and the State*. Oxford, Oxford University Press, 261–270.

Dubé L et al. (2014). From policy coherence to 21st century convergence: a whole-of-society paradigm of human and economic development. *Annals of the New York Academy of Sciences*, 1331(1):201–215.

Gellner E (1994). *Conditions of liberty: civil society and its rivals*. London, Hamish Hamilton.

Goldberg E (1996). Thinking about how democracy works. *Politics and Society*, 24(1):7–18.

Greer SL (2016). Who negotiates for a nation? Catalan mobilization and nationhood before the Spanish democratic transition, 1970–1975. *Democratization*, 23(4):613–633.

Greer SL, Lillvis DF (2014). Beyond leadership: political strategies for coordination in health policies. *Health Policy*, 116(1):12–17. doi: 10.1016/j. healthpol.2014.01.019.

Greer SL, Wismar M, Figueras J, eds. (2016). *Strengthening health system governance: better policies, stronger performance*. Maidenhead, Open University Press.

Habermas J (1975). *Legitimation Crisis*. Boston MA, Beacon Press.

Heinrich VF (2005). Studying civil society across the world: Exploring the thorny issues of conceptualization and measurement. *Journal of Civil Society*, 1(3):211–228. doi: 10.1080/17448680500484749.

Jensen MN (2006). Concepts and conceptions of civil society. *Journal of Civil Society*, 2(1):39–56. doi: 10.1080/17448680600730934.

Keane J (2013). *Civil Society: Old Images, New Visions*. Chichester, Wiley.

Kickbusch I, Gleicher D (2012). *Governance for health in the 21st century. A study conducted for the WHO Regional Office for Europe*.

Kirkpatrick J (1979). Dictatorships and double standards. *Commentary*, 68(5):34.

Kohler-Koch B, et al. (2013). *De-mystification of participatory democracy: EU-governance and civil society*. Oxford/New York, Oxford University Press.

Laurent-Ledru V, Thomson A, Monsonego J (2011). Civil society: a critical new advocate for vaccination in Europe. *Vaccine*, 29(4):624–628.

McQueen D et al. (2012). *Inter-sectoral governance for Health in All Policies: Structures, actions and experiences*. Copenhagen, WHO Regional Office for Europe on behalf of the European Observatory on Health Systems and Policies.

Malena C, Volkhart FH (2007). Can we measure civil society? A proposed methodology for international comparative research. *Development in Practice*, 17(3):338–352. doi: 10.1080/09614520701336766.

Mann M (2004). *Fascists*. Cambridge, Cambridge University Press.

Marmot M (2004). *The Status Syndrome: How Social Standing Affects Our Health and Longevity*. New York, Times Books.

Marmot M, Bell R (2012). Fair society, healthy lives. *Public Health*, 126, Supplement 1:S4–S10. doi: http://dx.doi.org/10.1016/j.puhe.2012.05.014.

Marmot M et al. (2010). Fair society, healthy lives: Strategic review of health inequalities in England post-2010.

Page E (2012). *Policy without politicians: bureaucratic influence in comparative perspective*. Oxford, Oxford University Press.

Parsons T (1975). The sick role and the role of the physician reconsidered. *Milbank Mem Fund Q Health Soc*, 53(3):257–78.

Pedahzur A, Weinberg L (2001). Modern European democracy and its enemies: the threat of the extreme right. *Totalitarian Movements & Political Religions*, 2(1):52–72.

Pilnick A, Dingwall R (2011). On the remarkable persistence of asymmetry in doctor/patient interaction: A critical review. *Social Science & Medicine*, 72(8):1374–1382.

Putnam R (1993). *Making Democracy Work: Civic Traditions in Modern Italy*. Princeton: Princeton University Press.

Trägårdh L, Witoszek N (2013). 'Introduction', in Trägårdh L, Witoszek N, Taylor B (eds.), *Civil society in the age of monitory democracy*. Oxford, Berghahn, 1–21.

Satyanath S, Voigtlaender N, Voth HJ (2013). Bowling for fascism: social capital and the rise of the Nazi Party. National Bureau of Economic Research.

Varshney A (2001). Ethnic Conflict and Civil Society: India and Beyond. *World Politics*, 53:362–398.

WHO (2012). *Health 2020: a European policy framework supporting actions across government and society for health and well-being*. Copenhagen, WHO Regional Office for Europe.

Chapter 2

What civil society does in and for health: a framework

Scott L. Greer, Monika Kosinska, Matthias Wismar

This chapter provides a framework, the matrix, for understanding the various types of organizations and activities of civil society with regards to health and health systems. This includes interest groups, professions, a large set of very diverse community-based organizations (faith, identity, locality, social and health-condition) and international non-governmental organizations. The types of activities include policy-making, service delivery and governance. These three activities are further subdivided in a total of eleven specific activities.

With this matrix, we map the territory we want to chart. We make the discussion on CSOs much more tangible by introducing sub-categories, we can demonstrate the great diversity and ubiquity of CSO and actions, and we hope that this matrix will be used in country work and cross-country comparison.

In what follows, this chapter will discuss in detail the matrix and the types of organization and action that engage for health and health systems.

This chapter builds on the preceding chapter, which set out the background of this study including our motivation, a definition of civil society, a discussion of what civil society can do for health and health systems, what are its principal instruments for engagement and where the limits of civil society are.

This chapter is followed by a concluding chapter which draws on the conceptual frameworks developed in Chapters 1 and 2 and summarizes the empirical evidence presented in Chapters 4 to 10 and the mini case studies.

2.1 The analytical matrix: types of organization and action

There are as many ways to classify CSO and health and health system-related actions, it seems, as there are CSOs and actions. Any classification could be made more specific or complete. Ours merely seeks to capture key types of civil society organizations that are found in different societies, and key types of action.

In some contexts, such as the European Union and many European states, there are detailed legal requirements and expectations for information about organizations, and penalties if the organization or its leaders deviate too far from what their legal situation requires. As a result it is possible to identify the workings of the organization in some detail. In most contexts, organizations have a means of self-identification, such as stressing their service or policy activities in their self-presentation.

This matrix, like the definition of civil society, is not meant to be exhaustive and is certainly not meant to incorporate all the gradations and variations in civil society and its status (for a similar but more nuanced version, see de Leeuw, (2015)). Rather, it is meant to identify types of civil society found in most societies, and the actions it exerts in most societies in relation to health.

This helps us to explain the place of civil society in health. Secondly, it provides some subcategories to better understand the large category of civil society. Thirdly, it identifies the great diversity and ubiquity of civil society and the kinds of activities that it performs in different places. This should enable cross-national conversations about civil societies by stressing that even if, for example, social partners and campaigning NGOs are quite different, they are both aspects of civil society. Fourthly, the matrix provides an analytical framework that can help us to discuss causalities or, in other words, what type of CSO might be the right choice for what type of action? We will not come up with a definite answer to this question as the case studies and mini case studies are rather exploring the matrix illustrating its usefulness. But we hope that it will help analysts, consultants and international agencies when discussing how governments can best work with CSOs. We also hope that it will inspire further cross-country comparison on CSOs and health.

2.2 Types of organization

There are three basic categories of organization that we use. Interest groups are united by a desire to promote a political interest. Community organizations exist for a reason that is not primarily political. Social partners are distinguished because they have a formal role in governance. A fourth category, international NGOs such as the Red Cross or Greenpeace, rates a mention simply because their context is made up of different kinds of interaction with many different kinds of society.

2.2.1 Interest groups

Interest groups are by far – and almost by definition – the most common kind of civil society representation in democratic politics. They are simply united by shared interests and values. They are CSOs that "sell" a cause, be it the influence of tobacco companies or the welfare of undocumented migrants. Political scientists typically insist on viewing all such groups as interest groups, since what is an altruistic and evidence-based cause in one person's eyes is a selfish and dogmatic intervention in politics in another's (and, in many cases, the self-interest of the organization's leaders in maintaining their stream of donations and invitations is a factor in organizational action).

We nonetheless divide between *business groups* and *causes*. Business groups are typically advocating for policies that benefit their members, while causes are advocating for policies whose benefits to donors and volunteers exceed the cost of advocacy. A pharmaceutical company might have a very clear financial incentive to support an interest group advocating for better patent protection, whereas there is little financial incentive for a person to donate to a charity (cause) focused on access to medicines in developing countries. A business interest group is one which is composed of or accountable to for-profit enterprises. It is therefore part of the market, rather than civil society, and we henceforth exclude business interest groups unless they are part of social partnership systems in which they are also legally accountable for broader interests in society. Chapter 9, in the case of Austria, shows how business associations can partner with unions and the state to govern health systems and the economy.

Interest groups of all kinds face the problem of free-riding. It is easy to let somebody else pay for representation of your shared interests. The way business interest groups operate is either by serving such a concentrated industry that the benefits of a given policy are clear and free-riding is hard, or by providing something else, a selective benefit such as insurance policies or information. Thus, for example, polluters have an incentive to club together and try to influence politics; the potential loss to their businesses from effective environmental regulation is greater than the cost of lobbying.

It is a truism of political science that in a free market for representation business will tend to buy the most representation. Businesses have money, relatively clear interests, and can identify the costs and benefits of participation in an interest group. Business lobbies consequently tend to dominate any political system, with more than four-fifths of lobbyists in the European Union and the United States. There is no homogeneous business interest, but there is a great deal of representation for most business interests (Greer, da Fonseca & Adolph 2008; Coen & Richardson, 2009; Mahoney, 2008; Eising et al., 2017). This means that lobbying expenses can be dramatic when there is a major dispute between industries such as pharmaceuticals and technology. It is also the reason why policing conflict of interest in civil society can be so important. Well resourced private sector lobbies will often see co-optation, or even creation, of grass-roots civil society as a reasonable strategy (the strategy of creating artificial grass-roots is sometimes called "Astroturfing" after a brand of artificial grass).

Economic groups of particular note include unions and trade associations, both of which can have roles as lobbies and as part of governance. Unions almost always have a mix of service and representational functions (although company or government unions, which often fail the test of autonomy, might have one or neither). When they are engaged in representing their workers before the government and negotiating for them before employers, they are interest groups. In systems with social partnership, however, unions or peak-level associations of unions can be tied in with employers' associations or peak-level employers' associations to jointly determine issues such as salaries, labour conditions, and employment rules. Likewise, a trade association with a simple representative function (such as lobbying the European Union) or a service activity (such as organizing an industry conference) is just an interest group. Only if it is involved in economic governance, normally by negotiating wages and labour conditions, is it a social partner.

Business interest groups are not, in our definition, part of civil society even though they are the numerically dominant form of interest group in most political systems. Causes-based interest groups are, however, a key part of civil society. They are the organizations that represent specific or general interests in politics, ranging from the most specific interest to the broadest issues of global welfare such as climate change. Cause-based groups are not accountable to or composed of for-profit enterprises. Chapter 4, about participation in the European Medicines Agency, shows how civil society organizations can be articulated with business lobbying in the very lobbyist-heavy EU environment.

2.2.2 Professions

Professions are the organizations representing and often self-regulating a set of professionals. They take forms such as medical associations and professional chambers. For our purposes we need not define professions to define professional organizations, but it is worth noting that professional organizations are no more the same as the profession than the group representing an ethnic group is an ethnicity (Greer, 2008). Professions frequently have a major role in governance, but in Chapter 7 we see how a Turkish medical society plays a major role in responding to the Syrian refugee crisis.

2.2.3 Community organizations

Communities are united by a shared identity that is not family and is not necessarily of the members' choosing; they are people who share a place or an identity of some sort, such as ethnicity, gender orientation, or a health condition such as being patients or having a specific disability. Communities are social groups united by a shared attribute. The organizations that represent and serve them, community groups, are our focus. Here we only discuss some of the most common and important, without disparaging other kinds of communities and civil society found among them. The different kinds of organizations that grow among them can then be evaluated for their combination of autonomy from state, market, and family, and for their representativeness of and service to that constituency.

2.2.4 Faith-based community organizations

Faith-based community organizations. Faiths can take in a wide variety of organizations, from large and relatively centralized to highly spontaneous and decentralized. Even when they are organized, it is not always clear how much power the hierarchy has, or how much ability to speak for its divines and practitioners of the faith. Nonetheless, the organizational dynamics of a faith are different from those of patients, an ethnicity, or a gender because the faith gives such coherence and connection, and channels both mobilizing potential and the kinds of commitment members will show. Organized religion has helped, for example, underpin collective responses to austerity in Cyprus (Chapter 6).

2.2.5 Identity-based community organizations

Identity-based community organizations are made up of people who share belonging to an ethnic or other group, typically through birth, and often with markers such as language, surnames, occupational or residential segregation, and cultural practices such as distinctive food or holidays relative to others in the society. They will sometimes also share a different religion, so in some cases the distinction between a religion and an ethnic group has little practical difference behind it. Ethnic communities will often have both service and policy organizations, and sometimes the same organization, such as a welfare organization, will supply both.

2.2.6 Local community organizations

Local community organizations are based in a locality, such as a neighbourhood or rural district. They can do work ranging from organizing village holidays to operating charities for the poor or representing their neighbourhoods in discussions about topics such as transportation and health care infrastructure. They are a variable rather than a constant. Some communities are well organized and some are not. Some have strong service organizations, some have strong representative organizations, some have both. Some have single big organizations, some have small and fragmented ones. What they have in common is that they serve or claim to represent an area. A local group's core interests and sphere of action is local, though they will sometimes have overarching regional or national organizations to coordinate local groups with shared ideas.

2.2.7 Social community organizations

Social community organizations are groups organized to enable some kind of social activity – anything from bird-watching to book clubs to singing to cooking to restoration of old cars. In most places the most common kind of social group is sporting clubs. Social groups have the least obvious link with health in many cases, but they are a big part of civil society (in some countries they are numerically overwhelming). It has been argued that even if social groups make no great claim to representation or service, the networks, connections, culture of joining and organizational skills that they produce strengthen the ability of civil society to carry out any function (Putnam, 1993). We do not have a specific chapter on them because most of the time their participation in health is indirect, improving health through empowerment, togetherness, sport, and friendship rather than through directly identifying and addressing health needs. That does not mean a strong social component of civil society is not a boon to health.

2.2.8 Health condition-related community organizations

Health condition-related community organizations (patient groups, support groups) (Löfgren, de Leeuw & Leahy, 2011; Baggott, Allsop & Jones, 2005; Strach, 2016). Condition-related groups, finally, are united by neither an ethnicity nor a faith nor a locale, but rather by a specific health attribute. We single them out from all the other potential ways to organize because of their special relevance to health. They can sustain civil society organizations that represent their interests, as with patients' rights groups, and also service work such as communities of knowledge and support for people and their families with particular diseases or conditions. Case study Eight, which is about a disability rights campaign in Bosnia, highlights the importance of health-related, including disability, groups for both advocacy directed towards society and mobilization of the members themselves.

2.2.9 International Non-Governmental Organizations

International NGOs are a category by themselves. Their size, visibility, international reach and distinctive funding and accountability relationships mean that they are only rarely comparable to NGOs that operate exclusively in the context of a single state.

2.3 Types of civil society activity

Like civil society and its organizations, the types of civil society activity are remarkably diverse and take different forms depending on social, legal, economic, and political context, as well as chance and individual entrepreneurship. It is nonetheless possible to identify some of the main types of activity in which civil society engages.

The core division is between *policy*, *service*, and *governance*. While many organizations do both, there is a useful distinction to be made between activities directed at influencing or making public policy and activities directed to provide a service, whether broadly for the public or specifically for members.

Policy means engagement in decision-making and public policy – representing interests, advocating for policies, pushing for implementation of decisions, challenging other decisions, and holding policy-makers to account in a watchdog capacity that enhances public sector accountability. *Service* means providing something directly, whether it is lottery tickets for casual buyers, subsidized hotel discounts for members, weekly football games for sporty locals, or a needle exchange for drug addicts. *Governance,* finally, is when civil society organizations have important social functions such as wage-setting or standardization delegated to them by public organizations. Many organizations, of course, do two or three of these and what they do can bring changes; for example, an apolitical football club might organize a political campaign, focusing on a single issue, to exert political influence, and become apolitical again as soon as the political aim has been achieved. if its grounds risk being built over, while a policy-focused organization might live off the revenue from magazine subscriptions or social events.

Table 2.1 *Actions and types of civil society organization*

Activity		Constituency									
		Interest groups			Communities					International	other
		Causes	Economic	Professions	Faith-based	Identity based	Local	Social	Health-related	International NGOs	Other
Policy	Evidence	(ch4)|(MC1)|(ch8)		(ch5)|(ch7)			(ch6)		(ch6)	(MC3)	
	Policy development	(MC1)|(MC4)	(MC4)	(MC4)					(MC4)	(MC3)	
	Advocacy	(ch4)|(ch8)					(ch6)		(ch6)|(MC7)|(MC8)	(ch4)|(MC3)	
	Mobilization	(ch4)|(ch8)|(MC2)|(ch10)		(MC5)			(ch6)		(MC5)|(MC7)|(MC8)		
	Consensus-building	(ch4)	(ch9)	(ch5)|(ch9)					(ch10)		
	Watchdog/ accountability	(ch10)|(ch4)									
Service	Services to members	(ch10)	(ch10)	(ch7)|(MC5)	(ch6)|(MC6)		(ch10)		(ch10)		
	Services to public	(ch7)|(ch8)	(ch10)	(ch5)			(ch10)|(ch6)|(MC6)		(MC5)|(ch10)	(ch4)	
Governance	Standards			(ch5)							
	Self-regulation			(h9)							
	Social partnership		(ch9)	(ch9)							

Source: Authors' elaboration

2.3.1 Policy activities

Influencing policy is best done all the time, since policy does not develop in stages and battles over the content of policy are not confined to one arena. Engaging in policy, though, involves a variety of different activities. Some organizations specialize more in certain kinds of activities and some political systems are more hospitable to one kind of activity than another.

Evidence and agenda-setting is the development and publicization of evidence on a topic of interest. This can mean, for example, asking members or conducting research on particular problems that the group would like to see addressed in public conversation and policy. It is sometimes rigorous and scientific, but will also often be resource-constrained and shaped by political context since it is not often judged by scientific standards and real social or biomedical research tends to be expensive. Often, bringing members' voices to the fore is one of the most constructive contributions that can be made. Thus, for example, we can see the evidence that the Russian anti-tobacco coalition as able to bring in the discussion in Chapter 4.

Policy development is engagement in a policy proposal from the "inside", through participation in formal structures such as consultative groups, public consultations, and lobbying. It means that a group is addressing policy-makers on their terms, discussing the agreed political agenda; that a group's ability to contribute is accepted by the key policy-makers; and that the group is playing by the established rules of the policy process. We see this throughout the book, particularly in the engagement of EU civil society organizations discussed in Chapter 4 and the influence of social partners discussed in Chapter 9.

Advocacy, by contrast, is engagement in policy from the "outside", addressing the public in order to foment social change or create pressure on the political system in order to shape policy.

Mobilization is close to advocacy but it is aimed at other people rather than at government. It goes beyond drawing attention to the issue and involves mobilizing people to act through techniques as diverse as petitions, demonstrations, membership drives and social media actions. Mobilization can also be directed at ends other than policy and engagement with the political system, such as mobilizing people to get screened for a disease or boycott a given product. In short, it is about changing the minds and actions of ordinary people rather than primarily persuading policymakers- though an organization that is good enough at mobilization will become more interesting to policymakers. Chapters 4 and 8, about tobacco and HIV/AIDS, both contain especially interesting examples of mobilization, as well as case studies 5 and 7, on hospice and obstetric care. In each case, changing minds is a major part of the work.

Consensus-building is a niche activity, but one that is found in many countries. It occurs when the political system is unwilling or incapable of formulating a consensus on an action but is willing to enact something presented as consensual. This kind of activity is often undertaken by scholarly associations with a political charter, but it can also be more participatory.

Watchdog work, finally, means monitoring public and private compliance with policy and ethics. It means keeping up the pressure after the policy is made so that organizations comply, new ministers are reminded to pay attention, and the penalties of non-compliance are felt (Tragårdh, 2013). This can involve research and publicity on non-compliance, administrative redress, and litigation, as well as leading to further advocacy (McLaren, 2015). It is an instrument of accountability that holds policy-makers responsible for implementing policies and decisions. The watchdog role of civil society is part of what makes the Dutch initiatives described in Chapter 10 so promising.

2.3.2 Service work

Service work, in contrast to policy work, delivers some kind of service to a specified population. Its finances can vary substantially, as will the type of organization. Political systems tend to homogenize interest groups – all the interest groups in a given polity tend to look relatively similar – but service organizations can reasonably range from tiny and local to huge and international. Evaluating them can be easier than evaluating organizations and initiatives whose goal is to change minds or policy, but still difficult and often possibly only over the long term.

Services to members. The first and probably most common kind of service is to members: religious services for members of a faith community, trade magazines for business associations, and matches for football players. These are simply services that require membership in the relevant community and probably in the specific CSO. The financial base of many CSOs will depend on selling such services, perhaps in order to finance other policy or service work.

Services to the public. Services to the public means the provision of services to people who do not make up the CSO or its core community; for example, disaster relief, needle exchange, and free medical care are all activities in which there is a distinction between the organizations and people providing the service, and those receiving it. CSOs are often densely concentrated in services to vulnerable, small, or difficult-to-reach parts of the public where governments cannot or will not engage effectively. We see examples in, for example, the Cypriot "social groceries" of Chapter 6, the aid to Syrian refugees in Chapter 7, and the assistance for people with HIV/AIDS in Chaper 8.

2.3.3 Governance

Sometimes civil society organizations play an explicit role in governance. There are three major areas in which we find civil society playing an explicit role: in technical standard-setting; in professional and other self-regulation; and in corporatist arrangements for governing the economy.

Standards. Standards underpin much of modern life, whether in the form of technology standards that enable the operation of key infrastructure and devices or in the form of organizational practices. Civil society organizations such as the International Standards Organization formulate more or less technical standards and thereby enable modern society and market competition to function. Within countries, there are many civil society standards organizations engaged in work as diverse as setting standards for road design, medical device interoperability, and good quality care for children. There is also a range of private standards organizations, for example the ones selling accreditation of health care providers (Jarman & Truby, 2013), but they are generally weaker because they are more problematic. Their profit motive introduces conflicts of interest and less sense of ownership, which gives them a harder task than that facing most civil society organizations.

Self-regulation. In many countries civil society organizations are responsible for a measure of self-governance. This is what distinguishes social partners, though it is not confined to them. It can mean, in many countries, that medical professional organizations take on the complex task of making, updating, and enforcing rules for good practice. It can also mean governance of the labour market, through economic tasks such as setting wages and working conditions (in which unions and employers negotiate sector-wide arrangements that are then enforced on and by their members).

Social partnership. Social partnership, also known as corporatism or neo-corporatism in the scholarly literature, refers to the organized representation of major parts of society, often as highly organized associations with peak leadership and economic and regulatory functions in the larger economy. There is a long tradition in many countries of assigning the "social partners" roles in the organization of society, with a governance role in issues such as wage-setting, working conditions, and workforce training (Schmitter, 1974; Streeck & Schmitter, 1991; Katzenstein, 1985). There is also a long tradition in even more countries of self-governing professions with responsibility for aspects of their members' professional competence and economic standing. The meaning and role of social partners and social partnership varies greatly over time and between countries, but their work can be very important in understanding how health systems operate and there are potentially valuable lessons for countries with less of a tradition of social partnership for managing health systems and policies. Social partnership is, broadly, associated with the world's most competitive and egalitarian economies, and countries with effective social partnership are the only ones to have weathered the post-2008 Eurozone crisis in good condition (Hancké, 2013), so it must have some serious advantages.

The key concept is social partnership, discussed in Chapter 9 with evidence from Austria: the idea that social partners, which are peak associations of employers and unions, have a role to play in shaping policy and engaging in direct governance. Without a basic *context* of social partnership, with a role for such corporatist governance, and organizations capable of mustering the participation and compliance of their members (firms, workers), then they are other kinds of civil society, especially interest groups. In some contexts, such as the EU, where there is little effective social partnership because there is no corporatist organization of the labour market, organizations that are social partners in their domestic context are recast as interest groups. Brussels, in this sense, is just not comparable to Member States because the odds of an EU-wide social partnership on the scale of a Member State ever developing are very slim. In other words: a profession, trades union, or employers' association is only a social partner in the context of social partnership that entrusts them with a role in governance. Otherwise they are interest groups.

2.4 Summing up the presentation of the matrix

This chapter has shown two things: first, that civil society takes many different forms; and secondly, that it does many different things. The options for partnership are therefore many, and policy-makers can partner intelligently with civil society in many ways. The options for partnership are therefore many, and policy-makers can partner intelligently with civil society in many ways. These options for partnership, however, are not arbitrary. It will be an empirical question to identify the best combinations of CSO and health actions. And this combination will depend a lot on regulative contexts and the instruments used in the government–CSO collaboration. These determinants of successful engagement with civil society will be presented in the next chapter, alongside a practical framework for health policy-makers wishing to engage with civil society.

References

Baggott R, Allsop J, Jones K (2005). *Speaking for patients and carers: Health consumer groups and the policy process*. Basingstoke, Palgrave Macmillan.

Coen D, Richardson J, eds. (2009). *Lobbying in the European Union*. Oxford, Oxford University Press.

de Leeuw E (2015). Intersectoral action, policy and governance in European Healthy Cities. *Public Health Panorama*, 1(2):175–182.

Eising R et al. (2017). Who says what to whom? Alignments and arguments in EU policy-making. *West European Politics*, 40(5):1–24. doi: 10.1080/01402382.2017.1320175.

Greer SL (2008). Medical Autonomy: Peeling the Onion. *Journal of Health Services Research and Policy*, 13(1):1–2.

Greer SL, Massard da Fonseca E, Adolph C (2008). Mobilizing Bias in European Union Health Policy. *European Union Politics*, 9(3):403–433.

Hancké B (2013). *Unions, Central Banks, and EMU: Labour Market Institutions and Monetary Integration in Europe*. Oxford, Oxford University Press.

Jarman H, Truby K (2013). Traveling for treatment: a comparative analysis of patient mobility debates in the European Union and United States. *Journal of Comparative Policy Analysis: Research and Practice*, 15(1):37–53.

Katzenstein PJ (1985). *Small States in World Markets: Industrial Policy in Europe*. Ithaca, Cornell University Press.

Löfgren H, de Leeuw E, Leahy M (2011). *Democratizing Health: Consumer Groups in the Policy Process*. Cheltenham, Edward Elgar Publishing Limited.

Mahoney C (2008). *Brussels versus the Beltway: Advocacy in the United States and the European Union*. Washington, D.C., Georgetown University Press.

McLaren ZM (2015). Equity in the national rollout of public AIDS treatment in South Africa 2004–08. *Health policy and planning*, 30(9):1162–1172.

Putnam R (1993). *Making Democracy Work: Civic Traditions in Modern Italy*. Princeton, Princeton University Press.

Schmitter, PC (1974). Still the Century of Corporatism? *The Review of Politics*, 36:85–131.

Strach P (2016). *Hiding Politics in Plain Sight: Cause Marketing, Corporate Influence, and Breast Cancer Policymaking*. Oxford, Oxford University Press.

Streeck W, Schmitter PC (1991). From National Corporatism to Transnational Pluralism. *Politics and Society*, 19(2):133–165.

Trägårdh L (2013). Associative democracy in the Swedish welfare state. In Trägårdh L, Witoszek N, Taylor B, eds., *Civil society in the age of monitory democracy*. Oxford, Berghahn.

Chapter 3

Working with civil society for health: policy conclusions

Scott L. Greer, Matthias Wismar

How can health policy-makers engage with civil society? This chapter brings together the discussion and case studies to formulate some basic policy conclusions. It integrates the discussion of civil society with the TAPIC governance framework, as discussed in other Observatory publications (Greer, Wismar & Figueras, 2016), focusing on ways in which governance and policy can contribute to effective civil society engagement in, and support for, health systems and policies. It first summarizes the case for working with civil society and developing appropriate tools to make that relationship fruitful, then discusses the basic regulatory framework that is necessary, and then introduces a practical framework for health policy-makers who wish to engage with civil society.

Box 3.1 *The TAPIC governance framework*

The TAPIC governance framework (Greer, Wismar & Figueras, 2016) identifies five key areas of governance that shape the decisions societies make and the way in which they are implemented. It is a diagnostic tool to identify and address policy failures and risks to effective policy that are attributable to governance, as against inadequate finance, lack of government backing, or impracticality. It has five components:

Transparency means that decisions and the grounds on which they are made are clear and public. It encourages civil society by allowing it to identify important decisions and opportunities.

Accountability means that actors are obliged to report their actions to clearly identified bodies such as legislatures which are able to sanction them. Making accountability clear and effective means that civil society can know which groups to target with information and advocacy.

Box 3.1 *contd*

Participation means that affected groups are able to participate in decisions even if they do not get to make the decisions. This means, above all, enabling civil society consultation.

Integrity means anti-corruption measures such as clear formal hiring processes, but also clarity in different organizations' roles. Civil society can promote this in a watchdog capacity and also benefits because corruption can exclude weaker, less wealthy, and less connected groups from policy-making.

Policy *capacity* refers to the resources available to governments to gather, understand and analyse information and formulate workable policies. Civil society can contribute with research and information that balances insider efforts, thereby diversifying government information at a low cost.

3.1 Civil society is ubiquitous, diverse, and beneficial

The first point of the book is that civil society is ubiquitous, diverse, and can be beneficial. Civil society in health is:

- *ubiquitous* and necessary because it exists, however informally, in all health systems and fulfils a role because there is always a place where markets, families and the state all fail to carry out some tasks or communicate. When people band together to do something, they are civil society. There is still great variation, and a few countries have curtailed the space for civil society and discouraged action, but it persists and those countries suffer from its absence.

- *diverse.* As our matrix and the case studies illustrate, there are many different kinds of civil society organization that do many different things, from local advocacy to European Union advocacy, and from organizing sport for local children to sharing in the governance of an entire country. Not all kinds of civil society are found everywhere, but even more exist than our matrix could show.

- *beneficial.* The ubiquity, energy, flexibility, efficiency and diversity of civil society mean that working with it is desirable, whether to provide services, improve policy-making and implementation, or to carry out governance functions.

Civil society is *not* some other things:

- Civil society is not a replacement for an effective public health system. Civil society organizations can deliver services on behalf of public systems, and they can sometimes raise money to fill gaps, but the same self-organizing and independent characteristics that make civil society valuable also make it insufficient to deliver universal health care. Some of the strongest civil societies are in countries that also have extremely effective publicly financed health care systems (Trägårdh, 2013) and in no country does charity finance anything resembling universal health care.

• Civil society is not a panacea for social ills. There is a great deal of positive writing about civil society, and this book emphasizes the benefits of a strong civil society for health systems. But civil society can also be divisive, reinforcing rather than bridging ethnic and other differences (Varshney, 2001) and it can become politicized and clientelistic, losing its autonomy to political actors or business.

• Civil society is not one thing. Its diversity, and the importance of context, mean that it is never wise to start out assuming that the nature of, and issues in, any given country's civil society are known, even to policy-makers in that country. Simple assumptions and language about the strength, weakness, and geography of civil society will fail (Ekiert & Kubik, 2014).

Civil society's role and activities are *not* guaranteed to take any given form:

• Civil society can be ineffective, corrupted, repressed, tamed, or a puppet for somebody else. This might be convenient for some interests, but it limits civil society's contribution to a broader society.

• Even if it is not, the diversity of civil society means that it is common for an officially designated civil society to be the formal face of the whole of civil society, limiting the benefits of hearing diverse voices and partnering with diverse organizations.

• The ubiquity of civil society does not prevent it having great variation in its size, strength, and vitality. The mere fact that people almost always organize something, somehow, does not mean that the persistence of amateur sports clubs, underground organizations, or traditional dispute resolution systems bespeaks a healthy civil society. Civil society might be almost everywhere, but it can be so weak as to hardly matter.

• Finally, civil society can be beneficial in health but that is not automatic. Benefits depend on a civil society that is indeed reflective of non-market, non-state, non-family interests in society, so not corrupted or instrumentalized but also strong and able to work in partnership with policy-makers.

The next section discusses the regulatory framework that is the baseline to have a civil society that can effectively and formally contribute to the health system.

3.2 Regulating civil society for health

First and foremost, not all civil society must be regulated. It should be up to a local advocacy group or soccer club or group of concerned citizens whether they want to be formally constituted as a group. Governments can create a wide variety of incentives for organizations to formally organize themselves, such as the ability to open bank accounts as organizations, beneficial tax treatment, or the opportunity to bid for government contracts. An incentive-based approach, rather than mandatory registration, is more effective, less costly, and less likely to stifle civil society.

Secondly, registration should not be made a hurdle. Not only does a complex registration process deter organizations that should be given a chance, it also creates the opportunity for officials to exercise discretion in political, corrupt, or other ways. The integrity of the bureaucracy may vary, but even in a government with a very high level of integrity there is still no reason to drag out registration, limited liability, and other procedures.

Thirdly, we should accept that there are gradients and variations in what kind of transparency and autonomy we can formally ask of civil society organizations. Conceptually, an organization is autonomous if it can select its own leadership, change its own rules, and make its own decisions even if that endangers its funding or status. In most cases, this can be made clear in its terms of incorporation. But as an organization becomes more important, such as through participation in government contracts or participation in policy-making forums, it is legitimate to ask for more information and specified behaviours such as, at a minimum, audited accounts or clear statements of funding sources. That is beneficial because it makes it less likely that government funds are wasted or participatory forums filled up with front organizations for some occluded interest. In cases such as fully fledged social partnerships (see Chapter 9), there is a very high degree of institutionalization of the social partners precisely because they are so integral to the way the health system, and the country, function. The capacity of governance in a country is important, too. If the civil service would be overstressed by registration requirements, or would be tempted to seek bribes as part of the regulatory process, then a lighter touch approach with simpler administration would be desirable.

Finally, and perhaps most importantly, the registration and handling of civil society organizations by government should be based in the rule of law, with very little administrative discretion. Government and government officials have many counterproductive incentives in dealing with civil society. They might want to colonize civil society in order to gain access to its jobs and resources; they might want to use it to build local political power bases; they might want its legitimacy to support whatever they want to do; they might want to block the formation and success of organizations with which they disagree; or they might want to discriminate against certain groups of people. The solution to all of these cases is to focus on clear rules with minimal administrative discretion. Basic registration, in particular, should have negligible government discretion. Otherwise, the risk is not just that government will stifle civil society, but that government officials will have far too many opportunities to manipulate it to personal ends that even their leaders would not approve.

Beyond these basic requirements, we did not find much of a case for further regulation of civil society. Civil society organizations should be made easy to found and operate precisely to gain the benefits of their diversity and experimentalism. It is reasonable to attach conditions to working with them, but those conditions should be clearly linked to public objectives such as preventing corruption and enhancing policy debate. A requirement that recipients of grants should not share expertise with government and the public, for example, is unreasonable since it cuts off government from knowledge and ideas while politicizing the handling of civil society.

3.3 Instruments for working with civil society for health

Once civil society's regulatory framework is constituted, there are many ways in which health systems can work with civil society. Following our matrix, we discuss some of the most common and important instruments for engagement in the areas of service, policy, and governance. As ever, it is worth remembering that civil society is diverse and its institutional contexts are also diverse. There is no one-size-fits-all model for engagement.

3.3.1 Service

Perhaps the most ubiquitous form of civil society engagement is in service provision. Civil society can respond, in many cases, faster than even the best organized states, as we saw with the social groceries in Cyprus (see Chapter 6), as well as in the UK (Loopstra et al., 2015) and Greece (Sotiropoulos, 2014), and with the refugee crisis in Europe that started to grow in 2014 (see Chapter 7). Civil society can reach out to relatively small groups, such as people with HIV who subdivide into quite different and internally diverse groups (sex workers, intravenous drug users, etc) (see Chapter 8). It will often be more effective for the government to support or contract with specific, sometimes very small, CSOs to address specific needs.

The two obvious ways for government to support service organizations are through contracts and grants. Contracts are ongoing business relationships built on payment for services rendered. A health system can contract with a CSO to run a care home or outreach service. Contracts naturally reduce the flexibility of the CSO, but can be highly effective for both parties. Grants are often responsive to CSO proposals and have less ex-post control since there is more ambiguity about what government is buying. They are therefore most common for relatively experimental tasks such as research where it is not so clear what the best possible endpoint will be. Both contracts and grants can allow civil society to expand and contract with need and enthusiasm; once Cyprus exits its crisis, there will be less need for the social groceries that Joachim discusses (see Chapter 6), and we doubt anybody will regret the diminished need.

In both cases, it is key that the government contracting process adheres to rules of good governance, in particular integrity and transparency. Otherwise there is immediate incentive to turn civil society organizations into fronts for political interests or something clientelistic and often to repress the more marginal interests that are best represented by civil society. This means, ideally, clear specification of broad objectives combined with regular feedback mechanisms and a legal procedure to prevent distortion of programmes and goals.

There are some more distinctive ways to support civil society, such as the religious tax that finances the large-scale charitable works of the German churches (which in turn were responsible for much of the response to the refugee influx of 2015) or various forms of tax deduction, effective most notably in the United States (where the donor gets the tax break) and in the UK (where donors can effectively grant recipients a tax break). It is less clear that these mechanisms can be exported to other countries, even though they are effective ways to give civil society autonomy from the state. To our knowledge nobody has tried the experiment of creating an American-style tax break for donations in a country with limited civil society – perhaps a statist tradition prevents both. There is not much evidence that tax codes actually shape the size and impressiveness of civil society – the US might be forgoing the tax revenue without getting a stronger civil society for it (Reid, 2017).

3.3.2 Policy

Civil society engagement in policy does not replace government but is highly advantageous. Civil society can represent views of different parts of society that might get drowned out in normal politics, even if civil society organizations almost never have the democratic legitimacy of an elected representative. For institutions which lack the direct legitimacy of a centuries-old state, such as the European Union, engagement with civil society can add to the legitimacy of their own policy-making and role. Precisely because the EU does not have a clear demos of its own, its institutions work to construct a European civil society that can inform its policy-making and improve its legitimacy (Schmidt, 2016; Jarman, 2011; Wincott, 2002; Kohler-Koch et al. 2013). This openness and desire to gain legitimacy for the EU from civil society participation has helped health advocates to shape EU policies (Franklin, 2016). Furthermore, interests will almost unfailingly make their preferences known – factions and interests are constants across all regimes. A structured form of engagement with civil society, just like lobbying, actually makes clearer the shape of politics, the affected interests, and the inequalities of power.

In choosing instruments for policy engagement with civil society, then, it is important to keep an eye on what civil society can bring, and the risks. The objective should be to create accessible forums that give government access to a diverse set of voices and ideas, while not biasing the process in favour of monied and other established interests that generally have good access to policy, and while being transparent about the ideas and interests in the debate. Thus, for example, patients associations have some potential to help address the problematic Cypriot health system (see Chapter 6) (Cylus et al., 2013) and similar problems in other countries (Rabeharisoa & O'Donovan, 2014).

Beyond this, there is an enormous number of specific tools, suitable to each culture and political system, that can allow for civil society participation in decision-making, and can make decisions transparent to civil society organizations. Common ones include:

- submissions to and testimony to legislative committees and hearings;

- advisory committees to individual ministers, departments, or agencies;

- structured consultations on decisions; and

- forums that engage a range of civil society organizations in discussion of policy challenges, such as the EU Health Policy Platform.

Each of these can be appropriate and useful in a given situation. Their functioning depends on details of design, their design and legislative base, and their political backing. The key thing for their designers is to focus on creating incentives for organizations to come with information and diverse and useful ideas and criticisms, and to avoid political bias or accidental bias such as towards organizations with extensive staff capacity.

The risk with civil society engagement in policy is that a lack of transparency and participation will bias the results. An intricate policy-making system, such as that found in the European Union, or one that confines formal engagement to a biased list of partners, as is often found in trade policy worldwide, is one that lobbyists for industry will be able to exploit better than any others. In such systems basic information becomes a challenge for organizations with other objectives such as environmental protection, access to medicines, or consumer rights. Opacity, complexity, and cost are all barriers that can be addressed. For example, if there are civil society forums, then the government should either use low-cost technologies (conference calls) for meetings or fund travel to meetings for representatives from groups with less money. Documents and data should not be published in needlessly complex format or rigid PDFs, but neither should they be reduced to infographics that cannot be interrogated by outsiders.

The risk is that policy-making becomes cumbersome, with lots of stages and regulatory barriers, but does not add real transparency or participation. The main negative consequence of costly opportunities to participate in opaque discussions will be a bias towards industry and a loss of the benefits of other civil society thinking and information. Such cumbersome policy-making creates major challenges to government capacity; civil servants need superb project management skills to shepherd legislation through in systems with multiple opportunities for participation. Policy-making should always therefore be sensitive to the need for clarity in proposals and support for broad civil society participation if the process is to produce high-quality information.

3.3.3 Governance

Civil society organizations that play a role in governance, as with social partnership or standard-setting, are performing public functions for the public good with state backing, and therefore need to exist in a world of more procedure, transparency, and institutionalization. There is a world of difference between the highly institutionalized social partners of Austria and an informal group for local advocacy or service. That is proper, since the Austrian social partners have far larger effects on many people's lives.

In creating social partnership, the definition discussed in Chapter 9 can serve as a guide. It involves authoritative organizations, such as the peak employers' and trades unions, an institutionalized structure that manages conflict and enables cooperation, and authority delegated from both public and private actors over key aspects of work such as labour regulation and wages. In many countries, social partnership is so established as to look like part of an overarching consensus culture, but other countries have achieved social partnership for longer or shorter times in order to, for example, join the European Union. What is key is to ensure that circumventing or seceding from social partnership will be a bad idea, by entrusting social partnership with authority in legislature, or by having strong peak employers' and unions' federations that can deter defection from the social partnership. Merely appealing to a concept of shared interests without creating any penalty for pursuing self-interest is unlikely to work.

In discussing more technical governance that is based on civil society, such as professional regulation and standard-setting, governments are even more directly delegating regulatory authority over a sector of the economy (even if they retain a final authority over each decision, which is common). In these cases, there are instruments such as charters that are effectively long-term contracts between the public authority and the civil society organization. Making the charter (of any organization, CSO or otherwise) revocable if the organization fails to fulfil its role is a distant but often effective enough means to ensure performance; and if worst comes to worst, the government can choose some other policy tool. In general, technical standard-setting happens in areas where the general interest is that a standard be set, but where everyone except the most directly interested parties is indifferent to the specifics. When the standards are starting to have broader effects on society and awaken broader interest, as with privacy or nanotechnology, governance based on civil society will often come under pressure. Likewise, as long as professional regulation works in the eyes of the public, it is an efficient and effective way for governments to ensure quality, but if public confidence is lost or the government starts to want a broader definition of quality, the regulatory system may quickly come under pressure, as happened in the UK (Salter, 2004).

3.4 A practical framework for health policy-makers engaging with civil society

Another way to put it is that policy-makers at any level who seek to engage with civil society for any health policy purpose – be it policy, delivery, or governance – can ask themselves the following questions. Answering each one is hard and requires work as well as thought, but the process can help guide policy.

1. Can you find civil society? This might seem like a simple question, but it is not. What are the key organizations in an area? For example, health managers might be unaware of the nature of civil society in an area until their proposals for service redesign cause a political firestorm. Policy-makers who want to work with vulnerable communities might not know which organizations already work with them. Ministries might be focused on only a few key interest groups and miss other groups with different perspectives. In each case, ignorance of civil society is the first problem.

2. Why are you engaging with civil society? Do you know what you want? This second problem reflects the diversity of contexts for both civil society and health policy. If the goal of engagement is to have innovative and flexible services, then one set of tools and skills, such as contracts, might be useful. If the goal is to gain input into policy-making, then another set will be

useful. Engagement for engagement's sake might be informative, but even if the goal is simply to build relationships, that should be made explicit.

3. Can/will civil society deliver? Does civil society want to deliver what a policy-maker seeks? Civil society varies enormously and the existing organizations might not have the capacity to do what is asked of them. A small service organization might be overwhelmed by the problem it is addressing. Groups in a given policy area might lack technical expertise or the resources to engage with government on the government's terms. Organizations that are supposed to be part of governance might lack resources or have conflicts of interest. Further, civil society organizations might not be positive about the policy or might not trust policy-makers enough to participate. In other words, ask whether the request is realistic.

4. Can you help civil society deliver? And can you be a better partner if they don't want to? If the problem is resources, then there are various ways to support civil society financially (and sometimes to reduce the cost of participation, e.g. through simpler consultation mechanisms). If the problem is disagreement, then patient engagement and trust-building might be necessary. All too often, health policy-makers only interact with civil society when it opposes them, and the result is that they meet on hostile terms. Knowing each other better might not lead to agreement, but at least it might lead to some measure of trust and knowledge.

5. Is time being managed appropriately? Consulting and working with civil society requires time for civil society to consult its own members, to make them understand the issues at stake, and to allow some measure of trust to build up. Engaging with civil society only in a crisis or oppositional context will make it difficult to engage constructively.

3.5 Conclusion

This study was inspired by Health 2020, the WHO European policy for health and well-being. Health 2020, in terms of policy-making, service delivery and governance, relies on intersectoral action. It is therefore promoting a whole-of-government and a whole-of-society approach. While the former focuses on cross-departmental cooperation inside government and administration, the latter, which is the subject of this study, encourages governments to reach out and engage with civil society.

This volume gives testimony to the need to consider and engage with CSOs when developing and implementing a Health 2020-inspired policy at country level.

This book's case studies show the diverse and impressive range of benefits to health systems and policies that come from listening to, working with, and even promoting civil society. The benefits might bring occasional frustration, but the same diversity and passion also means that policy-makers can hear additional voices, gain more buy-in to their decisions, deliver services quickly and responsively, and avoid immersion in unnecessary technical arguments. While the ubiquity of civil society shows that it is always necessary to modern life, policy-makers will often find that a well managed engagement with a healthy and diverse civil society will make health systems, policies, and societies better.

We were also aiming at providing orientation for students, consultants and policy-makers interested in civil society and health. We hope that the definitions, the matrix, including types of CSO and actions, will be of help in analytical terms. Addressing more practical issues, we hope that our discussion on regulation and instruments for civil society will be of help. The framework for engagement will hopefully stimulate debate in countries providing some of the nuts and bolts necessary for successful collaboration.

The case studies have demonstrated wide variations of dealing with civil society. Some countries embrace civil society and CSOs have become indispensable in health and health systems. Other have been more skeptical and have even curtailed in recent years the space for CSO. Therefore, for the Member States of the WHO European Region, – and the same is true on a global scale – a key challenge that will remain is to develop acceptance, contexts and regulation conducive to working together.

To many readers, a generally positive discussion of civil society might seem uncontroversial. But during this project, we saw the scale of the challenges surrounding the relationship between civil society and health policy-making. It is very tempting for policy-makers to ask what has happened when they give a grant to an organization which then criticizes them, as happens everywhere. It is very tempting for local politicians to turn a CSO into a political base and exploit it, as we often see in southern Europe. It is even more tempting when there is foreign funding for CSOs, as we have seen across much of central and eastern Europe. It is also, finally, tempting to just tolerate a minimum of civil society and try to sculpt it to particular ends. But such temptations should be resisted, for a healthy civil society and health system.

References

Cylus J et al. (2013). Moving forward: Lessons for Cyprus as it implements its health insurance scheme. *Health Policy*, 110(1):1–5. doi: 10.1016/j. healthpol.2012.12.007.

Ekiert G, Kubik J (2014). Myths and realities of civil society. *Journal of Democracy*, 25(1):46–58.

Franklin PK (2016). Public health within the EU policy space: a qualitative study of Organized Civil Society (OCS) and the Health in All Policies (HiAP) approach. *Public Health*, 136:29–34. doi: 10.1016/j.puhe.2016.02.034.

Greer S, Wismar M, Figueras J eds. (2016). *Strengthening health system governance: better policies, stronger performance.* Maidenhead, Open University Press.

Jarman H (2011). Collaboration and consultation: Functional Representation in EU Stakeholder Dialogues. *Journal of European Integration*, 33(4):385–399.

Kohler-Koch B et al. (2013). *De-mystification of participatory democracy: EU-governance and civil society.* Oxford/New York, Oxford University Press.

Loopstra R et al. (2015). Austerity, sanctions, and the rise of food banks in the UK. *BMJ*, 350:h1775.

Rabeharisoa V, O'Donovan O (2014). From Europeanization to European Construction. *European Societies*, 16(5):717–741. doi: 10.1080/14616696. 2014.946069.

Reid TR (2017). *A Fine Mess: A Global Quest for a Simpler, Fairer, and More Efficient Tax System.* London, Penguin Publishing Group.

Salter B (2004). *The New Politics of Medicine.* Basingstoke, Palgrave Macmillan.

Schmidt V (2016). Reinterpreting the rules 'by stealth' in times of crisis: a discursive institutionalist analysis of the European Central Bank and the European Commission. *West European Politics*, 39(5):1032–1052. doi: 10.1080/01402382.2016.1186389.

Sotiropoulos D (2014). Civil society in Greece in the wake of the economic crisis. *Report for Konrad Adenauer Stiftung und ELIAMEP.*

Trägårdh L (2013). Associative democracy in the Swedish welfare state. In Trägårdh L, Witoszek N, Taylor B eds., *Civil society in the age of monitory democracy.* Oxford, Berghahn.

Varshney A (2001). Ethnic Conflict and Civil Society: India and Beyond. *World Politics*, 53:362–398.

Wincott D (2002). The Governance White Paper, the Commission and the Search for Legitimacy. In Arnull A, Wincott D eds. *Accountability and Legitimacy in the European Union.* Oxford, Oxford University Press:379–398

Part II

Chapter 4

The Russian Anti-Tobacco Advocacy Coalition (ATACa)

Kirill Danishevskiy, Martin McKee

Editors' summary

This case study is about introducing and firming-up tobacco control policies and measures in Russia. Russia was chosen because after the collapse of the Soviet Union, the international tobacco industry was in a strong position to influence policies to their advantage. This chapter focuses on the health related Russian Anti-Tobacco Advocacy Coalition (ATACa). This case study demonstrates how civil society organizations can help shape government policy vis-à-vis powerful and relentless industry lobbies, by bringing (international) evidence to the table, provide advocacy, mobilization and act as watchdog. Moreover, ATACa established consensus among key civil society organizations. The chapter also illustrates how important the autonomy of civil society organization is, as all too often the tobacco industry tries to undermine the independence of institutions and officials. The case study also demonstrates that engaging with civil society requires at least transitional funding. The authors conclude that it seems likely that the changing view on the tobacco industry has played a part in the substantial decline of smoking rates in Russia.

The editors

For the transnational tobacco companies, the collapse of the Soviet Union was an unmissable opportunity (Gilmore & McKee, 2004a). At a stroke, they gained access to a market of 281 million people, 142 million of whom lived in the Russian Federation. Some 60% of Russian men were already smokers and the industry believed that it should be relatively easy to persuade them to shift to international brands. Smoking rates among women were much lower, at about 10% (Gilmore et al., 2004), but the industry's carefully crafted marketing techniques could be relied on to increase this figure, linking smoking to glamour and the perception of western sophistication (Gilmore & McKee, 2004b). Their task was facilitated in several ways. First, there was a hunger for foreign direct investment, often supported by western governments (Gilmore & McKee, 2004b). Secondly, there were many opportunities to take advantage of the inexperience and, in some cases, the greed of their counterparts in the countries concerned. Thus, in the absence of other sources of guidance, they could effectively write the rules on crucial issues such as taxation and tobacco control legislation (Gilmore, Collin & McKee, 2006). And, thirdly, unlike in western countries, there was no tradition of civil society organizations that could advocate for effective tobacco control policies. They were successful. At a time when smoking rates were falling in many western countries, the high rates among Russian men were maintained and those among women rose (Fig. 4.1).

Under the communist system, many of the organizations that would elsewhere comprise key elements of civil society, such as trade unions and professional, cultural and scientific bodies, were controlled by the party. In the 1980s some groupings had emerged, largely in areas where they were not perceived as a threat to the established political order, such as in relation to culture and the environment (Weigle & Butterfield, 1992). However, they were largely absent from the health arena. It was not until the aftermath of the transition, in 1991, that civil society organizations, as understood elsewhere, emerged. Among the most prominent were the Open Society (Soros) Foundations, established in

Fig. 4.1 *Trends in smoking prevalence in the Russian Federation during the early years of transition*

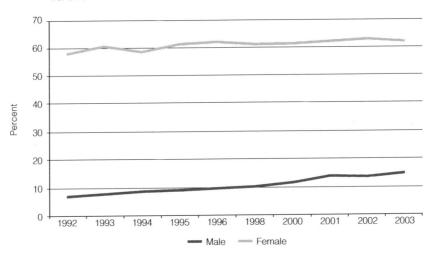

Source: Perlman et al., 2007.

countries across the region (Silova & Steiner-Khamsi, 2008). They operated across many sectors, including governance, law and justice, and the arts, but also, from the late 1990s, in health.

By the early 2000s these national foundations had become well established and in 2003 they were spun off into independent bodies. In the Russian Federation the new organization, now called the Open Health Institute (OHI), began operating in January 2003 with three years of transitional funding from the parent Open Society Foundations. It focused on two main activities. The first, on communicable disease, provided an extensive portfolio of harm reduction programmes designed to prevent HIV transmission, as well as a diverse set of small-scale activities, including alleviation of the often appalling conditions in prisons and pre-trial detention centres (Bobrik et al., 2005). The Harm Reduction programme had inherited significant co-funding from various international agencies, including the United Kingdom's Department for International Development. Following the spin-off, OHI established a consortium of five non-governmental organizations (NGOs) that attracted a large grant from the Global Fund against AIDS, TB and Malaria. The non-communicable disease programme was much less well endowed but ran initiatives in public health education, medical journalism, mental health, evidence-based medicine and palliative medicine, but these were not priorities for international donors and attracted hardly any co-funding.

Just before the transitional funding was about to end, OHI convened a strategic planning meeting to explore scope for the funding of non-HIV-related activities. Fifteen NGOs that were already partnering with OHI participated, each arguing for prioritization of different topics. The head of the "Healthy regions association" was a solitary voice arguing for tobacco control, and specifically to advocate for the Russian Federation to accede to the Framework Convention on Tobacco Control (FCTC). Over the course of four days he continued to make this case, in the face of strong opposition, based on a concern that such an activity could never attract funding in the Russian Federation. Moreover, those present recalled that OHI was already unpopular with Russian officials for promoting harm reduction, a policy that was opposed by many politicians who saw illicit drug use as primarily a matter for the criminal justice system. There were concerns that fighting the tobacco industry, linked to certain prominent politicians, could further jeopardize the status of the OHI. Eventually, a few OHI staff said that they would work, unpaid, for a few hours each day on a letter writing campaign, recruit *pro bono* external advice on dealing with tobacco lobbyists, and convene one or two press conferences under the auspices of the Medical Journalism programme. However, few thought that this would develop much further.

The results far exceeded expectations. After a few months, in August 2006, a National Coalition of seven NGOs "For Russia's accession to the WHO Framework Convention on Tobacco Control" was established. The coalition sought to unite the efforts of the leading community organizations striving to protect the health of the nation with the primary aim of promoting FCTC accession. Within three months more than 3,000 letters were written, to parliamentarians and public officials, calling on the Russian Federation to accede to the FCTC. Nikolay Gerasimenko, head of the Duma's (parliament) Health Committee, participated in OHI's media activities and initiated the first large-scale Health and Tobacco conference in the Russian Federation. Inevitably there were clashes with representatives of the tobacco industry but, for the first time in the Russian Federation, the health advocates won the debates.

Unexpectedly, four months after commencing these activities, Michael Bloomberg announced a Global Initiative to Fight Tobacco; one of its first grants, of $770 000, was awarded to OHI. This enabled it to create an even wider anti-tobacco coalition, the Anti-Tobacco Advocacy Coalition (ATACa).

Box 4.1 *The objectives of ATACa*

- Preparation and dissemination of information related to current trends in tobacco smoking, and the tactics used by tobacco companies, as well as actions to de-normalize smoking and decrease its prevalence.
- Increasing understanding of the harm associated with tobacco smoking by the population and health care providers.
- Providing and supporting a high level of coverage in the mass media related to the preventability of diseases caused by tobacco smoking in Russia, and the actions of the industry aimed at promoting smoking and undermining tobacco control, as well as the need for effective responses by governmental authorities.

This was established in August 2007, with the additional support of the International Union for Tuberculosis and Lung Diseases Control. Its goals were to support effective measures for tobacco smoking control and promote the Russian Federation's accession to the WHO FCTC. The coalition soon attracted many established NGOs, with more than 15 coming together by the end of the first year of the project (Box 4.2). The coalition grew rapidly from the activities of a few enthusiasts working in their free time, rather like Don Quixote tilting at windmills, to become a powerful movement posing an appreciable threat to previously unchallenged Russian tobacco company affiliates. Media engagement had formed a core part of ATACa's strategy (Box 4.3). The Bloomberg grant enabled a considerable scaling-up of this activity. Media coverage supportive of tobacco control increased from one or two

---

Box 4.2 *Current members of the Coalition (as of 1 December 2008)*

1. Open Health Institute
2. International Confederation of Consumers' Societies
3. All-Russian non-governmental organization "The League of patients' protection"
4. Regional non-governmental organization "Healthy Regions Association"
5. Union for struggle for public sobriety
6. All-Russian community movement "Sober Russia"
7. Russian philanthropic Foundation "No to Alcohol and Drug Abuse"
8. Foundation of Social Development and Public Health "FOCUS MEDIA"
9. Coalition "For Tatarstan free of tobacco smoke"
10. Russian Public Health Association
11. Cochrane Collaboration
12. Arkhangelsk International School of Public Health
13. Interregional non-governmental organization "Society of evidence-based medicine specialists"
14. Interregional non-governmental organization "Assistance to public health"
15. Non-profit partnership "Parental meeting", city of Ulyanovsk
16. Philanthropic foundation "Open Medical Club"
17. Non-governmental organization for a sober and healthy lifestyle "The Nizhnekamsk optimalist"
18. Association of University Programmes in Healthcare Administration

---

Box 4.3 *Media activity*

- A large number of press conferences and workshops on tobacco control were organized for journalists, covering many different parts of the country (Moscow, St Petersburg, Perm, Kazan, Tver, Stavropol, Arkhangelsk and Sochi).
- A training course for journalists was delivered, entitled "Public health: business, the state and society".
- A distribution list has been compiled of journalists working in the mass media (TV, radio, printed and electronic publications).
- The programme has reached out to regional media, with over 130 media events taking place on the subject of tobacco control (publications and interviews in the mass media, participation in TV and radio programmes, etc.).
- A project web site (www.ataca.ru) has been maintained, with additional support for pages on tobacco control on the web sites of coalition partners.
- A web site has been developed to expose tactics used by the industry to market tobacco products to young people and adolescents.

publications to between 25 and 50 publications per day with an accompanying improvement in the quality of the discourse, including polling evidence showing that there was widespread support for much stronger tobacco control measures than were being considered (Danishevskiy, Gilmore & McKee, 2008). Indeed, after the first year it was difficult to find a politician who was not informed about tobacco control and, specifically, the Framework Convention, with many openly talking about it.

When the grant proposal was being drafted, international experts providing *pro bono* support had discouraged the inclusion of Russia's accession to the FCTC as a Key Performance Indicator, seeing it as hopelessly ambitious in the time available. Yet, within one year, on 24 April 2008, the Russian Federation acceded to the FCTC. This was achieved by a multifaceted strategy involving the media (Box 4.4) and identification of an engagement with key stakeholders at the

---

Box 4.4 *Monitoring studies*

ATACA has undertaken a series of monitoring studies to assess the extent to which existing tobacco control legislation is being implemented.

It conducted a survey to ascertain whether there were any tobacco outlets within 100 metres of children's, educational and sports facilities in the territories of Bogorodskoye (Eastern administrative district) and Orekhovo-Borisovo (Southern administrative district) in Moscow. Such outlets were then illegal under Federal law #87-FZ "On the limitation of tobacco smoking". A number of violations were observed and the information was provided to the Federal Consumer Protection Service, the Moscow government, the prefectures of the administrative districts and the Central Moscow Department of Internal Affairs.

More than 2,000 measurements were taken of the quality of ambient air in 50 of the premises of major Moscow cafeteria and restaurant chains. In those that had failed to implement comprehensive smoking bans, the amount of tobacco smoke in non-smoking areas was only 24 per cent lower, on average, than in smoking areas. Thus, while in the smoking area about 30 cigarettes are smoked per hour, customers in non-smoking areas inhale an amount of smoke comparable to what would have been present if they had been in a smoking area where about 23 cigarettes were smoked each hour. Even when rooms were quite separate, with extra ventilation, there was no significant decrease in the amount of tobacco smoke. In some chains the level of air pollution in non-smoking areas was similar to measurements obtained in the Lefortovo tunnel (third Moscow transport ring, under the Yauza river) during the rush hour (when the speed of the traffic does not exceed 10 km per hour). However, in the "Coffee Bean" chain, where a total smoking ban had been introduced, the air did not contain any tobacco smoke. The results were subsequently published in the mass media.

federal level. For example, considerable effort was put into awareness raising, with participation in meetings and conferences, and organization of round table discussions at the Federation Council and the State Duma of the Russian Federation, the Public Chamber, the Moscow State Duma, *Rospotrebnadzor* (the authority in charge of consumer protection and public health), and *Roszdravnadzor* (the authority responsible for supervision of medical facilities and ensuring compliance with health legislation), on controls on the production and consumption of tobacco products. This was complemented by a campaign of letter writing, aimed at key decision-makers, including the President and Prime Minister of the Russian Federation, the Chairman of the State Duma and the Council of the Federation, the heads of various committees, deputies and senators, ministries and departments. In total, more than 700 letters were sent. In addition, several open letters were published in the mass media, including an appeal to the Mayor of Moscow in *Moskovskaya Pravda* in April 2008 and an appeal to the Chairman and the deputies of the State Duma in *Rossiyskaya gazeta* in November 2008.

Consistent with the approach taken by tobacco control advocates elsewhere, the importance of tackling the industry head-on was recognized from the outset. Thus, the Coalition acted as a spoiler at industry events. It undertook regular monitoring of public hearings in Parliament and industry involvement with the authorities and the media. Legislative initiatives by the pro-tobacco MPs were a particular focus, ensuring that the views of the tobacco companies were challenged. Such events were frequently attended by well trained ATACa speakers, arguing effectively against the industry's agenda.

Recognizing the global nature of the struggle against the tobacco industry, ATACa established an International Advisory Board, comprising Professors Anna Gilmore and Martin McKee from the United Kingdom and Dr Elizabeth Van Gennip from the Netherlands. The Advisory Board was able to facilitate the exchange of experience with other countries on tobacco industry tactics and how to combat them.

Although many of the activities were focused at the federal level, regional initiatives were not ignored, taking advantage of the existence of a number of regional public health and anti-tobacco organizations. For example, in Tver region a non-governmental organization, "Healthy Regions Association", organized a two-day training workshop for journalists in the region, a conference for teachers devoted to teenage smoking, at which effective and ineffective measures related to child and adolescent smoking were discussed, and a regional conference on "Health or tobacco" with the participation of physicians, teachers, scientists, and representatives of the Tver region and city administration. These activities have had a lasting effect. Even though they were initiated almost a decade ago, several of them continue even now, with the participation of the federal Ministry of Health.

Other regional activities were undertaken in Arkhangelsk, with the support of the governments of the Nordic countries; in Stavropol, supported by the regional government; in St Petersburg, supported by Oxfam; and in Kazan and Perm, with the support of the organization "Campaign for the future without cigarettes".

Local activity also involved the creation of demonstration projects, such as support to the Moscow City Centre for Tobacco Smoking Prevention and Treatment, at the Narcological Dispensary Clinic #9, which includes a free telephone hotline for help in smoking cessation.

The most important objective of ATACa was to achieve a decline in smoking rates. It can be reported that this has been achieved, with rates falling substantially in the Russian population, as revealed by two surveys undertaken within the framework of the project (Table 4.1). Clearly these changes cannot be attributed in their entirety to the work of ATACa. However, it seems likely that the changing views on the tobacco industry that the project promoted are likely to have played some part.

Table 4.1 *Prevalence of smoking among adults in two surveys conducted in November 2007 and May 2009 within the framework of the project*

Round of survey	Gender (%)		Both genders (%)
	Male	**Female**	
Proportion of smokers, November 2007	64.0	18.9	39.3
Proportion of smokers, May 2009	58.8	18.2	36.6

At the time of writing (2017), ATACa is still operating. There is still much to do. From its early days, ATACa has highlighted the anomalous situation whereby the Russian Criminal Code prohibits the sale or production of goods which do not meet established safety criteria, or which cause harm to health. Tobacco is clearly such a product, killing 50 per cent of those who use it as intended. Moreover, Russian law makes no exemptions for tobacco, or for any other goods already on the market that are later found to be harmful. Although the challenges are enormous, the ATACa coalition continues to campaign for tobacco to be treated like any other dangerous substance. While many might feel that the chances of success are extremely low, so, it seemed at the time, was the quest to get the Russian Federation to accede to the FCTC. In other words, nothing is impossible.

References

Bobrik A et al. (2005). Prison health in Russia: the larger picture. *Journal of public health policy*, 26(1):30–59. doi:10.1057/palgrave.jphp.3200002.

Danishevskiy K, Gilmore A, McKee M (2008). Public attitudes towards smoking and tobacco control policy in Russia. *Tobacco control*, 17(4):276–283. doi:10.1136/tc.2008.025759.

Gilmore A et al. (2004). Prevalence of smoking in 8 countries of the former Soviet Union: results from the living conditions, lifestyles and health study. *American journal of public health*. 94(12):2177–2187.

Gilmore AB, Collin J, McKee M (2006). British American Tobacco's erosion of health legislation in Uzbekistan. *BMJ* (Clinical research ed.), 332(7537):355–358. doi:10.1136/bmj.332.7537.355.

Gilmore AB, McKee M (2004a). Moving East: how the transnational tobacco industry gained entry to the emerging markets of the former Soviet Union – part I: establishing cigarette imports. *Tobacco control*, 13(2):143–150.

Gilmore AB, McKee M (2004b). Tobacco and transition: an overview of industry investments, impact and influence in the former Soviet Union. *Tobacco control*, 13(2):136–142.

Perlman F et al. (2007). Trends in the prevalence of smoking in Russia during the transition to a market economy. *Tobacco control*, 16(5):299–305. doi:10.1136/tc.2006.019455.

Silova I, Steiner-Khamsi G, eds. (2008). *How NGOs react: Globalization and education reform in the Caucasus, Central Asia and Mongolia*. West Hartford, CT, Kumarian Press.

Weigle MA, Butterfield J (1992). Civil society in reforming communist regimes: The logic of emergence. *Comparative Politics*, 25:1–23.

Case study 1

Together for a tobacco-free society: Slovenia

Vesna-Kerstin Petrič

In the last 20 years Slovenia has made substantial progress in tobacco control, becoming one of the "five countries in Europe that were able to reduce smoking prevalence below 25% for the adult population" (Gro Harlem Brundtland, WHO ministerial conference in Warsaw, 2002).

As a consequence of this success, in early 2000 there was little pressure for adopting stricter measures. Civil society was mostly represented by non-smokers' associations that operated on small grants and failed to form coalitions to advocate for the introduction of additional tobacco control measures.

In 2001 the Ministry of Health established a new department for health promotion and public health focusing on risk factors, including tobacco control. The Ministry became a partner in an international initiative that was launched in Central and Eastern Europe in 2000 by the Cancer Society from the USA (https://www.cancer.org/about-us.html), the Advocacy Institute, Washington DC (http://www.advocacyinstitute.org/index.shtml) and the Maria Sklodowska-Curie Cancer Centre & Institute of Oncology, WHO Collaborating Centre for Tobacco Control (http://www.who.int/tobacco/about/partners/collab_centers/poland/en/). The initiative involved government, press, medical professionals and NGO representatives from Central and Eastern European countries developing a campaign, based on the Great American Smoke-out. The campaign aimed at building coalitions and strengthening in-country advocacy capacities.

Based on this experience, and encouraged by the processes supporting the adoption and implementation of the Framework Convention on Tobacco Control (FCTC)[1], the Ministry of Health started to invest in NGOs' capacity building, prioritizing those which had established active cooperation with international networks, such as the European Network for Smoking Prevention (ENSP) and the Union for International Cancer Control (UICC).

The Slovenian Coalition for Public Health, Environment and Tobacco Control (SCTC), involving 26 NGOs, was founded in 2003 and became an official member of ENSP in 2006 and of UICC in 2009

(SZOTK, http://zadihaj.net/english/). In addition, in 2006 the No-Excuse youth organization was established (http://www.noexcuse.si/about-us), which developed a network of young tobacco control activists, implemented peer to peer projects for schoolchildren and published a Slovenian version of the Young people tobacco manifesto (http://ec.europa.eu/health/archive/ph_determinants/life_style/tobacco/help/docs/manifesto_en.pdf). No-Excuse contributed to the work of several international youth networks such as the Alcohol Policy Youth Network, the European Environmental and Health Youth Coalition, Sustainaware – Global Youth Partnership for Education on Sustainable Development, YU-SEE and the Tobacco Control Youth Network.

These two organizations took an active part in the public debate in 2007 when Slovenia was in the process of adopting a total smoking ban in public places and raising the smoking age limit to 18 (http://www.pisrs.si/Pis.web/pregledPredpisa?id=ZAKO471#). Their strong advocacy skills and good access to media were key to the successful adoption of the law. Both organizations remain active to date and in 2017 were significantly contributing to the adoption of a new tobacco law in Slovenia, introducing *inter alia* a total ban on advertising, donation and sponsorship; plain packaging; and licensing (http://www.pisrs.si/Pis.web/pregledPredpisa?id=ZAKO6717 ref).

Reference

[1] WHO Framework Convention on Tobacco Control. World Health Organization (2003), updated reprint 2004, 2005; http://www.who.int/fctc/text_download/en/).

Chapter 5

Engaging with civil society: the successful example of the European Medicines Agency

Ilaria Passarani[1]

Editors' summary

This case study is about introducing patient and consumer representation in the regulatory process of the evaluation, supervision and safety monitoring of medicines. The UK based European Medicines Agency (EMA) was chosen as an example because of its outstanding importance for the EU pharmaceutical market including the industry, payers, citizens and patients. This chapter focuses on the involvement of CSOs, which are mainly health related, economic or represent professions. This case study demonstrates how civil society organizations can provide evidence, help build consensus on decision making and contribute to standard setting. They improve the governance by improving the overall quality of the decision making process and the quality and transparency of science based decision making. The case study also demonstrates that civil society participation adds to the credibility of the processes, the decisions and the institution itself. It shows the benefits of participation of CSOs in decision making. To facilitate orderly CSO engagement regulation was drafted and funding was secured. The authors concluded that this

1 Declaration of interest: Ilaria Passarani works as Head of the Food and Health Department at the European Consumer Organization BEUC. Ilaria is also a member of the European Medicines Agency (EMA) Management Board and of the EMA patients and consumers working party. The views expressed in this chapter are personal and do not reflect the position of BEUC nor of EMA.

long standing structured engagement between EMA and patients and consumers' organization is the key to successful NGO participation.

The editors

5.1 Introduction

The European Medicines Agency (hereafter EMA or Agency) is a decentralized agency of the European Union. It was established in 1995 and it is responsible for the scientific evaluation, supervision and safety monitoring of medicines available on the EU market.

Over the last 20 years EMA developed a comprehensive framework for interaction with civil society organizations (hereafter CSOs) to improve scientific discussions on medicines which ultimately result in better outcomes of the regulatory process.

The CSOs dealing with EMA are mostly patients and consumers' organizations, health care professionals' associations, the pharmaceutical industry and academia. This chapter focuses on CSOs representing patients and consumers. First, it provides an overview on CSO involvement in the regulatory process from a theoretical perspective and describes the research methods. Secondly, it explains how the collaboration began and how it is currently working in practice. Thirdly, it offers concrete examples of the main factors that facilitate the engagement of CSOs. It concludes with an analysis of the added value of CSO involvement in regulatory decisions.

5.2 CSO involvement in the regulatory process

According to Everson & Vos, the BSE crisis of the 1990s and the consequent loss of credibility of the EU risk governance system triggered "institutional and procedural reforms to ensure the quality and transparency of science-based decision making and an invitation to citizens to participate throughout the process" (Everson & Vos, 2009, p. 1). From the institutional perspective, this led to the clear separation between risk assessment and risk management and the creation of independent scientific bodies like the European Food Safety Authority and the European Medicines Agency. From the procedural point of view, this was reflected in greater openness and transparency of the regulatory process and greater public involvement.

The involvement of citizens and CSOs is aimed at improving both the overall quality of the decision-making process and the quality of the scientific opinions. CSO input contributes to the knowledge base of decision-makers by enabling "lay knowledge to be introduced into the process of the production of 'hard science knowledge'" (Everson & Vos, 2009, p. 8). In this context, for regulators, CSO knowledge has both an instrumental and a legitimizing function (Boswell, 2009b), while CSOs provide knowledge to influence the decision-making process and align the belief system of regulators to their own.

Confronted with complexity, uncertainty, and bounded rationality, regulators involve CSOs to gain legitimacy and credibility. Feldman & March (1981, p. 178) state that, "using information, asking for information, and justifying decisions in terms of information have all come to be significant ways in which we symbolize that the process is legitimate, that we are good policy-makers, and that our organizations are well managed". Majone (1998) defines two dimensions of legitimacy: a procedural dimension and a substantive dimension. Procedural legitimacy implies that the institutions have been created by a democratically enacted legislation which defines their legal authority and objectives, that their employees are nominated by elected officials and that their policy-making process follows well defined procedures, which usually define the opportunity and the rules for various interest groups to be involved in the policy-making process; procedural legitimacy also refers to the fact that any decision must be justified, monitored, and open to judicial review. The substantive legitimacy refers to the level of expertise of the regulators, their capacity to protect public interests, the ability to choose the right priorities, and the capacity to ensure consistency between their activities and their stated objectives. Scharpf (1997) distinguishes between input-oriented and output-oriented legitimacy. Input legitimacy refers to the functioning of organizations and the procedures by which decisions are made and the capacity to align decisions to the preferences of people as a result of citizens' participation. Output legitimacy refers to the performance of the organization in relation to the quality of the final decision and the extent to which the outcome of the decision-making process caters to the public interest.

Legitimacy also arises from the support of CSOs and from CSO understanding of the work of regulators. Inspired by the Chinese proverb "Tell me and I will forget, show me and I will remember, involve me and I will understand", Kaza portrayed the need for stakeholder involvement as "with involvement comes understanding, with understanding comes public support and commitment" (Kaza, 1988, p. 76).

5.3 Research methods

The study is based on a review of the literature on knowledge utilization theories

(Heclo, 1974; Weiss, 1979; Lindblom, 1990; Radaelli, 1995; Boswell, 2009a), informational lobbying theories (Crombez, 2002; Broscheid & Coen, 2003; Coen & Richardson, 2009; Chalmers, 2013), and theories of the policy process (Sabatier, 1988; Majone, 1992). Data were gathered from documents of the European Medicines Agency and of the EU institutions and from participant observation. Gold (1958) suggested a typology of observational methods making a distinction between the possible roles of the researcher based on how much they participate in the field of the study. On one side of the scale there is the complete participant and on the other side the complete observer. In classic ethnographic studies the researcher is somehow in-between, while in this specific study the author can be considered as complete participant. Complete participation includes reflexive insider accounts. There is a tradition of sociological autobiography where personal experiences are used for research purposes. In these cases, experiences become data only retrospectively, and, at the time they are made, there is no intention to use them analytically for research purposes. What distinguishes ethnography from common sense is that it is not merely an insider description, but also an outsider analytical view. The author had a privileged direct observation of EMA engagement with CSOs as a representative of the European Consumer Organisation (BEUC) in EMA activities. Because of this, the observation of the field investigated was in principle done on a daily basis and it is difficult to quantify the number of relevant events observed. By approximation the most relevant experiences could be identified as the following: 40 meetings of the Patients and Consumers Working Party (four meetings a year from 2006 to 2016), 2 meetings of the EMA scientific advisory group on vaccines, 3 meetings of the EMA management board, 20 EMA conferences and workshops, review of 48 EMA information material for the public, and response to 16 EMA consultations.

5.4 EMA and CSOs

5.4.1 A long tradition of collaboration

EMA has been engaging with CSOs since it started its operations. The push came from both sides. On the CSO side, HIV patients' groups were among the first to encourage EMA to open towards civil society and engage with CSOs. In particular, in 1996 they provided input to the Agency on the value of surrogate markers in the approval of anti-HIV medicines leading to the early approval of protease inhibitors. On the Agency side, in the same year, the Management Board acknowledged that the partnerships between regulators and the "customers" are "at the heart of the regulatory system. If any of them were weakened or fractured in any way, the effectiveness of the system would be threatened" (EMEA[2],1996, p. 7).

Over the years, the interaction was also supported and formalized by legislators. With the legislation of orphan medicines that came into force in 2000 (Reg. (EC) 141/2000)[3], patients were appointed for the first time as members of one of the scientific committees of the Agency, namely the Committee for orphan medicinal products. The Regulation governing the functioning of EMA adopted in 2004 (Reg. (EC) 726/2004) requires the Agency to develop contacts with the Agency's stakeholders (Art. 78) and foresees that representatives of patients are appointed as members of the Management Board (Art. 65). The EU legislation also foresees that representatives of patients' organizations are appointed as members of the Paediatric Committee (Reg. (EC) 1901/2006, Art. 4), of the Committee for Advanced Therapies (Reg. 1394/2007, Art. 21) and of the Pharmacovigilance and Risk Assessment Committee (Reg. 1235/2010, Art. 61a).

In May 2002 the Agency organized the first workshop with patients and consumers' organizations which led to the establishment, in 2003, of a working group with eight patients and consumers' organizations. Building on the experience of the working group, in 2005 EMA developed a formal framework of interaction with patients and consumers' organizations. The framework included a clear definition of patients and consumers' organizations, the criteria to be fulfilled by CSOs willing to take part in Agency activities, and the creation, in 2006, of the EMEA working party with patients and consumers' organizations (PCWP).

The patients and consumers' organizations engaging with the Agency represent both disease-specific patients' organizations, such as the European AIDS Treatment Group and the European Cancer Patient Coalition, as well as general patients and consumers' organizations, such as the European Patient Forum and the European Consumer Organization.

Over the years the relationship with CSOs evolved substantially, not only in relation to the number of CSOs involved but also in terms of frequency and structure.

Fig. 5.1 outlines the overall number of patient and consumer involvement in EMA activities between 2007 and 2015. According to EMA's 2015 annual report, the sharp increase between 2014 and 2015 is partly due to the creation of topic groups established to brainstorm and make recommendations on topics of mutual interest between the Agency and the CSOs.

---

2 From 1995 unril 2009 the Agency was called the European Agency for the Evaluation of medicinal products. In 2009, following the adoption of a new organizational structure and visual identity, the Agency also changed its name and acronym into the European Medicines Agency (EMA).

3 Recital n.6. http://eur-lex.europa.eu/LexUriServ/LexUriServ.do?uri=OJ:L:2000:018:0001:0005:en:PDF.

Fig. 5.1 *Overall number of patient and consumer involvement in EMA activities (2007–2015)*

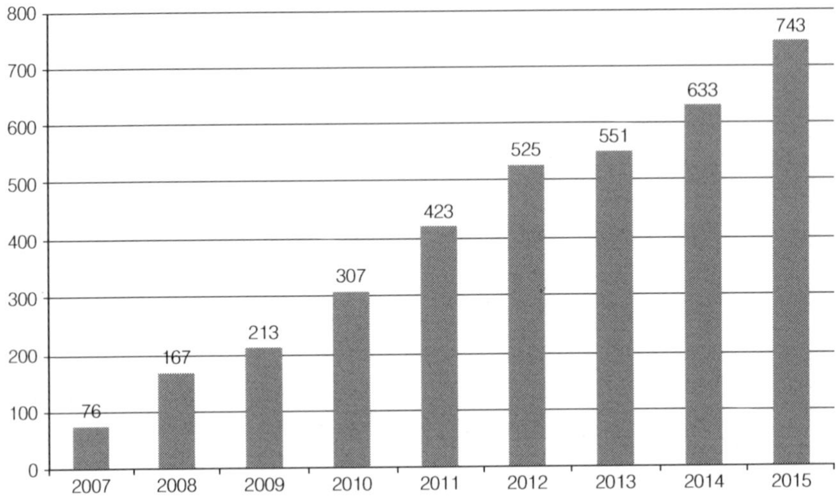

Source: EMA, 2015.

5.4.2 General principles, activities, and tools

Building on the experiences of many years of collaboration, in 2016 the Agency developed an overarching framework to manage the relations with all its stakeholders. The framework outlines the fundamental principles on which the interaction is based, namely independence and integrity, transparency, accountability, appropriate interaction, broad representation, effective communication, and continuous improvement. It also identified four levels of CSO involvement: inform, consult, consult and involve, cooperate/participate (EMA, 2016).

Patients and consumers' representatives take part in many EMA activities, most of which are channelled via the patients and consumers working party (PCWP). The PCWP serves as the main forum of exchange between EMA and CSOs. It meets four times a year and it is co-chaired by the Agency and by a representative of CSOs elected by the working party. The mandate, objectives, and working methodology of the PCWP, as well as the full list of its members and the minutes of all meetings, are publicly available on the Agency web site (EMA, 2013).

Within the PCWP, patients and consumers represent their own organizations and provide recommendations to the Agency on various topics that are relevant for patients in relation to the use of medicines, such as information, pharmacovigilance, rational use, and clinical trials. They also contribute to Agency consultations (e.g. EU network strategy to 2020, consultation of the pharmacovigilance and risk assessment committee on risk minimization strategies for medication errors with high strength and fixed combination insulins) and regularly participate in Agency workshops (e.g. workshop on shortages, workshop on adaptive pathways) and conferences.

As individual experts, they review written information on medicines prepared by the Agency, such as package leaflets, European Public Assessment Report (EPAR) summaries, and the Agency safety communications to the public, to ensure they are understandable by a lay person. For example, in 2015 they reviewed 137 of these documents. In addition, they bring the patient perspective into scientific advice and protocol assistance procedures and into the Agency's Scientific Advisory Groups (SAGs).

Lastly, as representatives of patients' organizations, they formally sit as members of the Management Board and several scientific committees (see also above).

The main tools used for CSO engagement are face-to-face meetings, a secured information system called Eudralink for the exchange of confidential product-related information (e.g. review of package leaflets for products that are not yet authorized), conference calls, workshops, trainings, and EMA staff participation in conferences and other meetings organized by CSOs.

From EMA annual reports it emerges that the collaboration with CSOs has significantly improved over the years and that both EMA and the CSOs made a great effort to make this collaboration effective and valuable for both sides.

The satisfaction questionnaires made by the Agency confirm that both EMA scientific committees and CSOs value the interaction positively.

5.5 Factors contributing to a successful collaboration

The main factor that has made the EMA–CSOs collaboration successful so far is their mutual interest in the collaboration. Patients and consumers' organizations have an interest in the activities of the Agency because they have a direct and indirect impact on the daily life of their constituency (such as access to medicines, safety, and information). The Agency needs patients' real-life experiences to improve understanding of the diseases and of the use of medicines. It also needs patients' and consumers' input to be able to communicate more effectively with the public.

The interaction is formalized both in EU legislation and in EMA documents. The official framework for interaction clarifies the roles of CSOs and the mutual expectations in relation to the results of the collaboration. The interaction with

CSOs is fully integrated in Agency work, including in its annual work plans and long-term strategy.

Another essential element that makes the interaction successful is the significant amount of resources allocated to implement the collaboration. This includes EMA staff entirely dedicated to the involvement of CSOs and the creation, in 2014, of a specific division responsible for public engagement, as well as a dedicated budget to cover all the expenses related to the organization of meetings and the travel expenses of CSO representatives to participate. It should also be noted that CSOs receive a daily allowance for participation in EMA meetings and that CSO representatives who work as volunteers for their organization receive a double daily allowance.

Other facilitating factors are transparency and clear rules. There is an open permanent call for expression of interest for CSOs who are interested in being involved with the Agency. A list of all the organizations which work with the Agency is published on the EMA web site. The CSOs must meet specific eligibility criteria which include: the legitimacy of the organization, which should have statutes registered in the EU; the organization's mission and objectives, which should be clearly defined; the activities of the organization, which should document a specific interest in medicines; the level of representation of patients and consumers across the EU; governing bodies elected by their members; accountability and internal consultation modalities; and the transparency of the sources of funding (EMA, 2014).

There are well defined policies about conflicts of interests and confidentiality that are the result of a consultation with CSOs and that guarantee CSO involvement while maintaining the integrity of the regulatory process. The EMA policy on handling conflicts of interest also allows patients' organizations that receive funding from pharmaceutical companies to take part in its activities provided the funding is diversified (where funding received from pharmaceutical companies exceeds 20% of the organization's total funding, this must be from at least three separate companies and the individual contribution from a single company should not reach the majority of the organization's total funding), transparent (the organization's financial accounts have to be published on its web site), and regulated by a code of conduct on relations with, and independence from, the pharmaceutical industry. However, when acting as representatives of their organization, patients and consumers are not allowed to participate in product-specific deliberations of the scientific committees. Patients acting as individual experts are subject to the same rules of conflict of interest as all other experts in the scientific committees. A three-layered policy on handling competing interests allows patients with links to the pharmaceutical industry (e.g. in a consultancy role) to bring their experience as patients without taking part in the deliberations of the scientific committee. In particular, on the basis of the information provided by the CSO representative, the Agency assigns a level of interest on the basis of the nature of the interest, the type of activity the CSO representative has to be involved in, and the time since the interest occurred. The CSO representative's participation is then restricted accordingly. CSO representatives are also required to sign a confidentiality undertaking, to abide by the Agency code of conduct, and to formally commit to taking an active role in the interaction with EMA.

Another key element of success is the regular monitoring of the CSOs both in qualitative and quantitative terms and the reporting of the interaction both internally (to the PCWP, to the scientific committees and to the Management Board) and externally with detailed annual reports published on the Agency web site.

Every two years EMA also conducts a survey via a perception questionnaire seeking CSOs' views on their interaction with the Agency, covering their satisfaction in relation both to the type of involvement and to the practical arrangements such as the organization of meetings.

Once a year EMA organizes a training for CSOs on the regulatory system in order to increase CSO knowledge of the EU regulatory process and of the work of the Agency, thereby facilitating involvement.

Another key element is the provision of feedback. The Agency usually provides feedback to CSOs with regard to the impact of the input they provided. This increases the perception that the input provided by CSOs is valued and taken into account. For many of the activities the impact of CSO collaboration is clearly visible. For example, out of the 47 EPARs summaries reviewed, 33 were amended as a result of patients' input (EMA, 2015).

The co-chairing of the PCWP and the consideration of CSO representatives as peer experts in the scientific committees increase the sense of ownership by CSOs.

The meetings are well prepared in advance with provision of the agenda and background documents. An individual and targeted preparation is offered to patients who participate as individual experts in a scientific committee. EMA also drafted a practical guide for patients visiting the Agency, which includes useful information, from administrative procedures to information about the facilities and equipment available.

Lastly, it should be noted that the interaction of EU umbrella organizations has a cascade effect because the CSOs involved in the Agency's activities disseminate the information to, and seek feedback from, their members, who are mostly composed of national associations or individual patients. This guarantees that information from EMA is spread more widely and that the input EMA receives from the patients and consumers' organizations is based on a larger constituency.

The highly technical level of EMA activities and the fact that the working language is English only can be considered as a hindering factor for an even wider involvement of CSOs. Moreover, the significant amount of time required to take part in EMA activities can discourage small CSOs with limited staff resources. From the Agency side, another hindering factor is the need to maintain the integrity of the scientific decisions. The main challenge is to combine the rigour of the evidence from clinical trials and post-market surveillance with the values and emotions of those who need the medicines. Another hindering factor for the Agency is the need to keep the collaboration manageable in terms of the number of CSOs it can interact with.

5.6 Legitimacy, transparency and trust: the added value of CSO involvement

The main tasks of the European Medicines Agency are to evaluate pharmaceutical companies' applications for marketing authorization, to monitor the safety of medicines across their lifecycle, and to provide information about medicines mostly to patients and health care professionals. The involvement of CSOs is essential to complement the assessment of the data gathered in clinical trials with real-life experiences of those affected by the diseases. This results in a more accurate evaluation of the benefit/risk profile of a product before and after it enters the market. With regard to the provision of information, EMA provides scientific information which is not easy to understand by a lay person. The involvement of CSOs helps the Agency to communicate more effectively with patients, contributing to the safe and rational use of medicines. In other words, CSO involvement is used to complement the knowledge base of the Agency, which comes mainly from purely scientific data, with the lay knowledge of the end users of medicines.

The Agency seeks knowledge from CSOs to improve the quality of its work and substantiate its scientific opinions, while CSOs offer their experience as patients and expertise as patients' representatives to promote their main interest, namely ensuring better access to safe and innovative medicines and high quality information. In this context knowledge has a substantiating function.

However, following scandals in the pharmaceutical sector – like the one concerning the weight-loss drug Mediator[4] which was linked with more than a thousand deaths in France (2011) and the more recent anti-vaccination

4 http://www.thelancet.com/journals/lancet/article/PIIS0140-6736(11)60862-3/abstract

movement – which challenge the work of regulators, the Agency also seeks CSOs' knowledge as a source of legitimacy.

As stated above, CSO involvement improves the quality of EMA scientific decisions and therefore contributes to the EMA mission, which is to foster scientific excellence in the assessment of medicines for the benefit of public health (output legitimacy). From an ethical point of view, patients have the right to be involved in decisions which are likely to have a significant impact on their daily life and on the health of many future patients. Their involvement helps to align EMA decisions with the preferences of those mostly affected by them (input legitimacy).

The well defined framework of interaction and the clear rules for CSO involvement in the decision-making process bring the Agency procedural legitimacy, as intended by Majone (1992). The engagement of CSOs also contributes to the Agency's substantive legitimacy as it improves its capacity to act in the interest of public health and achieve its main objective, i.e. enabling patients to access safe treatments.

The legitimacy also derives from the increased knowledge among CSOs about the regulatory process as a result of the trainings organized by the Agency, and from direct CSO involvement in many of its activities. Overall, CSO participation increases the transparency of the regulatory process and reinforces CSO and public trust in EMA's work.

5.7 Conclusions

CSOs formally and effectively contribute to the activities of the European Medicines Agency. They bring the Agency the unique perspective of those who are using or going to use the medicines that EMA evaluates and monitors, leading to a better outcome of the regulatory process and a better protection of public health. CSO involvement increases the understanding of how medicines are assessed and how the regulatory system functions, and at the same time increases the transparency of the process. This improves public trust in the Agency and the quality of the scientific decisions.

The structured form of interaction between EMA and patients and consumers' organizations is the result of many years of collaboration and constant improvement and can be used as a model for other bodies willing to engage with CSOs. It can be considered as a successful example of engagement as it brings benefits both to the Agency and to CSOs. It provides concrete measurable results which indicate that CSO involvement is not just a cosmetic exercise but an integral part of the work of EMA.

References

Boswell C (2009a). *The political uses of expert knowledge: Immigration policy and social research.* Cambridge, Cambridge University Press.

Boswell C (2009b). Knowledge, Legitimation and the Politics of Risk: The Functions of Research in Public Debates on Migration. *Political Studies*, 57:165–186.

Broscheid A, Coen D (2003). Insider and Outsider Lobbying of the European Commission. An Informational Model of Forum Politics. *European Union Politics*, 4(2):165–189.

Chalmers AW (2013). Trading information for access: informational lobbying strategies and interest group access to the European Union. *Journal of European Public Policy*, 20(1):39–58.

Coen D, Richardson J (2009). *Lobbying the European Union: Institutions, Actors, and Issues*. Oxford, Oxford University Press.

Crombez C (2002). Information, Lobbying and the Legislative Process in the European Union. *European Union Politics*, 3(1):7–32.

EMA (2013). Patient Health Protection Mandate, objectives and rules of procedure for the European Medicines Agency Human Scientific Committees' Working Party with Patients' and Consumers' Organisations (PCWP), 30 May 2013. EMA/369907/2010 Rev. 2.

EMA (2014). Stakeholders and Communication Division, Evaluation of financial information from patients', consumers' and healthcare professionals' organisations for assessment of EMA 'eligibility', 12 June 2014, EMA/566453/2012.

EMA (2015). European Medicines Agency's interaction with patients, consumers, health care professionals and their organizations. Annual report 2015.

EMA (2016). Stakeholders and Communication Division, Annual report on EMA's interaction with patients, consumers, healthcare professionals and their organisations (2015), 16 June 2016 EMA/727872/2015.

European Agency for the Evaluation of medicinal products, Second General Report, 1996.

Everson M, Vos EIL (2009). *The Scientification of Politics and the Politicisation of Science*. In Everson M, Vos E eds., *Uncertain Risks Regulated*. London, Routledge/Cavendish Publishing, pp. 1–17.

Feldman MS, March JG (1981). Information in Organizations as Signal and Symbol. *Administrative Science Quarterly*, 26(2)(June):171–186. London, Sage Publications.

Gold R (1958). Roles in sociological field observation. *Social Forces*, 36:217–223.

Heclo H (1974). *Modern Social Politics in Britain and Sweden*. New Haven, CT, Yale University Press.

Kaza S (1988). Community Involvement in Marine Protected Areas. *Oceanus*, 31(1):75–81.

Lindblom CE (1990). *Inquiry and Change. The Troubled Attempt to Understand*. New Haven, CT, Yale University Press.

Majone G (1992). Europe's 'Democratic Deficit': The Question of Standards. *European Law Journal*, 4:5–28.

Majone GD (1989). *Evidence, Argument and Persuasion in the Policy Process*. New Haven, CT, and London, Yale University Press.

Radaelli CM (1995). The role of knowledge in the policy process. Journal of European Public Policy, 2(2):159–183.

Regulation (EC) No 1901/2006 of the European Parliament and of the Council of 12 December 2006 on medicinal products for paediatric use and amending Regulation (EEC) No 1768/92, Directive 2001/20/EC, Directive 2001/83/EC and Regulation (EC) No 726/2004.

Regulation (EC) No 726/2004 of the European Parliament and of the Council of 31 March 2004 laying down Community procedures for the authorisation and supervision of medicinal products for human and veterinary use and establishing a European Medicines Agency

Regulation (EU) No 1235/2010 of the European Parliament and of the Council December 2010 amending, as regards pharmacovigilance of medicinal products for human use, Regulation (EC) No 726/2004 laying down Community procedures for the authorisation and supervision of medicinal products for human and veterinary use and establishing a European Medicines Agency, and Regulation (EC) No 1394/2007 on advanced therapy medicinal products.

Regulation No 141/2000 of the European Parliament and of the Council on orphan medicinal products.

Sabatier P (1988). An advocacy coalition framework of policy change and the role of policy-oriented learning therein. *Policy Sciences*, 21:129–169.

Scharpf FW (1997). *Games Real Actors Play. Actor-Centered Institutionalism in Policy Research*. Boulder, CO: Westview.

Weiss CH (1979). The many meanings of research utilization. *Public Administration Review*, 39(5):426–431.

Case study 2
Working with society to reduce corporal punishment of children in Finland

Maria D. Ramiro González and Dinesh Sethi

Corporal punishment is a serious threat to a child's well-being and development, and its use in societies is associated with higher levels of child maltreatment (physical, emotional, sexual abuse and neglect). The UN Convention on the Rights of the Child enshrines the right to a safe and violence-free life. The government of Finland banned corporal punishment in 1984, but in view of concerns about its persistence, the Ministry of Social Affairs and Health in Finland developed the National action plan to reduce corporal punishment of children 2010–2015, Don't hit the child![1] This was also in response to civil society groups such as the Central Union for Child Welfare (CUCW), an umbrella organization of non-governmental organizations (NGOs) and other stakeholders.[2] This influential advocacy group successfully supports the implementation of projects in this field in coordination with several NGOs.

Among these, the Federation of Mother and Child Homes and Shelters has a project that promotes positive parenting and awareness about children's rights and the ill-effects of violence.[3] The target groups are families, children, parents, adults and professionals related to child care and welfare. Families are supported to manage their daily lives and to strengthen parent-child interaction. They have raised awareness on the ill-effects of violence and every child's right to a non-violent childhood. The Family Federation of Finland is another NGO working to provide support for families with preventive activities related to childhood and parenting.[4] They offer internet services including online lectures, discussion boards, real-time chat boards, groups and informative videos on parenthood. Carers who feel challenged by the responsibility of parenting can seek expert guidance and mutual support from others. Their web site receives about 26 000 visitors every month. Another NGO, Miessakit Association, works on supporting fatherhood.[5] The goal of the project is to improve parenting in fathers, to disseminate good practices and training.

These three NGOs have worked successfully to implement the Finnish National action plan to reduce corporal punishment of children and have the support of the Ministry of Social Affairs and Health. The

Finnish experience shows how strong civil society advocacy and close working in parallel with legislative and policy change has improved child-rearing and reduced corporal punishment.

References

[1] Don't hit the child! National action plan to reduce corporal punishment of children 2010–2015. Available online: https://julkaisut. valtioneuvosto.fi/handle/10024/72278, accessed 16 June 2017.

[2] Central Union for Child Welfare. Available online: https://www. lskl.fi/english/, accessed 16 June 2017.

[3] Federation of Mother and Child Homes and Shelters. Available online: https://ensijaturvakotienliitto.fi/en/, accessed 16 June 2017.

[4] Family Federation of Finland. Available online: http://www. vaestoliitto.fi/in_english/family_services/, accessed 16 June 2017.

[5] Miessakit Association. Available online: https://www.miessakit.fi/ en, accessed 16 June 2017.

Chapter 6

Civil society, resilience, and participation in times of austerity: the case of Cyprus

Maria Joachim

Editors' summary

This case study is about strengthening civil society mobilization to a population in need. Cyprus was chosen as an example as it was particularly hard hit by rising unemployment and austerity policies as a consequence and response to the financial and economic crisis. The chapter focuses on a large variety of CSOs and their social activities, including the provision of basic goods and setting up of social groceries to assist individuals and families, demonstrating how local civil society organizations can respond in delivering timely services to the public. In addition, this chapter demonstrates how an existing organization such as the Pancyprian Federation of Patients' Associations and Friends has taken a leading role in representing patient organizations and advocating for health system reform under labour market and austerity conditions which exacerbated the health system's existing challenges. The author concludes that the positive experiences from CSO engagement during the crisis has led to strengthening resilience and participation of civil society within and outside health in Cyprus.

The editors

Since 2012 Cyprus has responded in several ways to the labour market changes and austerity measures which followed as a result of the financial crisis and the island's bailout from the Troika in 2013. These conditions strengthened civil society mobilization, highlighting it as an example of resilience amidst the mistrust that many Cypriots feel towards the government and their future. As such, civil society activities have been instrumental in supporting individuals and families both physically through the provision of basic needs as well as psychologically through social solidarity. In addition, while individual patient association groups in Cyprus continued, and still continue, to function as they did prior to the financial crisis, the presence of the Pancyprian Federation of Patients' Associations and Friends, an umbrella organization representing all patient groups in the country, has grown tremendously stronger in advocating for patients' rights and patient participation in decision-making after the financial crisis.

The following chapter aims to offer insights about how civil society in Cyprus has successfully responded to labour market changes, the financial crisis, and austerity, especially with respect to patient and health matters. **Section 6.1** provides an overview of the Cypriot social welfare system, **Section 6.2** discusses the labour market and austerity as they have impacted society in Cyprus, and **Section 6.3** illustrates how the Cypriot government and the private sector have been advocating the spirit of volunteerism and working with civil society. **Section 6.4** shows how labour market challenges and austerity have given rise to civil society resilience in the Cypriot society, and lastly **Section 6.5** provides a brief summary of the health system in Cyprus and explores the ongoing changes and efforts of a new health champion organization that advocates for patients' rights and stronger patient participation in decision-making and policy-making in Cyprus.

6.1 Cyprus: society and the social welfare system

Prior to 1974, social expenditures represented a small proportion of Cyprus's Gross Domestic Product (GDP). However, the Turkish invasion in 1974 and the Greek-Cypriot refugees – no less than 40% of the total Greek population of Cyprus at the time – created urgent social problems that needed to be addressed by the state. As a result of the invasion, as well as in alignment with guidelines for social welfare and social rights in other EU Member States, the Cypriot welfare state has gradually developed into a relatively complex net of social benefits and publicly provided social services. Essentially, the Cypriot welfare state developed into three parts: social insurance, universal protection and social assistance. The general social insurance scheme (GSIS), administered by the Ministry of Labour, Welfare and Social Protection, is compulsory and funded by contributions made by the working population, employers and the state.

The GSIS is designed to protect the working population against certain risks such as unemployment, illness, and disability. Universal protection provides income benefits to all households that satisfy certain criteria irrespective of their income. The most notable examples of universal protection include the child benefit given to all families according to family income and number of children in the family and the student grant given to families with children pursuing tertiary education in Cyprus or abroad. Social assistance provides a safety net to families that lack sufficient economic resources to support themselves (infoCyprus, 2016b; Koutsampelas, 2011). In addition to social security, the most important taxes levied and collected by the central government in Cyprus are income tax, value-added tax and corporate tax. Income taxes are levied on a progressive rate with the current brackets varying from 0% below €19 500 to 35% for salaries in excess of €60 000 (PWC, 2014).

Incentives for high salary, job stability and numerous benefits in the public sector during active employment years as well as after retirement have traditionally made the public sector very attractive for the Greek-Cypriot citizen. Employment in the broad public sector in Cyprus over time has included employment in the general government sector and in publicly owned enterprises and companies, making up about 42% of the total working population prior to the financial crisis (Eurofound, 2008). It is also worth noting that Greek-Cypriots have traditionally saved a big proportion of their salaries to guard against future emergencies, as well as for their children's education. In addition to a predominant culture of saving, the interest rates on savings accounts in Cyprus had historically been as high as 7% in the 1980s and 1990s, thus encouraging the population to practise saving, with families able to have cumulative saving deposits of over €100 000.

6.2 Labour market and austerity: changes for society and health

While the Cypriot labour market was characterized by high employment rates and low unemployment for many years leading up to the global 2008/2009 financial crisis, the severe worsening of those macroeconomic conditions resulted in rapidly rising unemployment with the debt-to-GDP increasing from about 49% in 2008 to 109% in 2013. It is estimated that overall unemployment (15–75 years) is currently 14.3% while youth unemployment (under 25 years) is at about 32.8% (Eurostat, 2015). In addition to increased unemployment, it is worth noting that the high interest rates of up to 7% on deposits in the previous decades have decreased significantly over the last five years with the current levels being around or below 2%. Many families now live in poverty while many households are on the verge of bankruptcy. This is especially the case for young individuals who have recently been able to establish a home and a family only to find themselves unemployed and unable to pay their home loans and day-to-day expenses.

As a result of the sovereign debt crisis in 2013, the Economic Adjustment Programme (EAP) for Cyprus was formally agreed by the government of Cyprus and the Troika in May of the same year. The EAP included a €12.5 billion bailout, including a €2.5 billion bilateral loan from Russia, in return for Cyprus agreeing to close the country's second-largest bank, Cyprus Popular Bank, also known as Laiki Bank. Depositors with savings less than €100 000 in Laiki Bank had their accounts transferred to the Bank of Cyprus, the largest bank on the island (Traynor et al., 2013). With regards to the Bank of Cyprus, the EAP imposed a one-time bank deposit levy of 47.5% on all deposits above €100 000 (also known as a bail-in of depositors), as opposed to the complete wipe-out in Laiki Bank. This was the first time that the euro-zone had made bank customers contribute to a bailout. In the case of both banks, no deposits of €100 000 or less were affected, while deposits over €100 000 were predominantly held by many wealthy Cypriot citizens or depositors from other countries, predominantly Russian nationals, who over the years had used Cyprus as a tax haven (Osborne & Moulds, 2013). In addition to the deposit levy, restrictions were imposed on withdrawals and on money transfers out of the country for many months.

As expected, the deposit levy caused uproar among the general public and ordinary savers. The bail-in created an elevated resentment and highlighted inequities between many families whose savings were a result of labour instead of avoiding taxation like many elite families. At the same time, ordinary savers were upset because precisely those elite families predicted the final bailout enactment and took action to transfer their deposits abroad into foreign banks before the bank levy and bank restrictions were implemented.

In addition to the bank levy and withdrawal restrictions, a Memorandum of Understanding (MoU) consisting of numerous fiscal and social welfare recommendations for the Cyprus system were agreed upon. Expenditure measures included reforms such as pension reform, reducing the number of public employees by at least 450 between 2012 and 2016, recruitment of one person for every five public sector retirees, and reduction of social transfers by at least €113 million through the abolition of different (often overlapping) schemes such as maternal allowances, wedding allowances, family allowances and educational allowances, as well as the special Easter allowance for pensioners. The MoU additionally required not only a freezing of wage increases in the public sector but also a scaled reduction in emoluments of public and broader public sector pensioners and employees as follows, ranging from 0.8%–2% according to salary (Ministry of Finance, 2013). Revenue measures, in addition to the deposit levy, included increased recommendations for increasing contributions to the GSIS, taxes on tobacco, beer and oil products.

6.3 Organizing civil society and participation

In 1973 the Pancyprian Welfare Council was created to provide information on CSO activity in Cyprus. In 2006 the council was renamed the Pancyprian Coordinating Council for Volunteers (Παγκύπριο Συντονιστικό Συμβούλιο Εθελοντισμού; PSSE) and has since served as an information platform for volunteers and volunteer organizations in Cyprus wishing to subscribe to the council as members. The Council's President is the First Lady, Mrs Anastasiades. In response to the increasing role of civil participation during the last few years, Cyprus has also established the first week of December as a "Volunteering Week", while the 5th Annual Convention on Civil Society was held in October 2015. In addition, since 2010 the council has organized an annual civil society conference. The latest of the five conferences, which was also held in October 2015, took the theme "Relationships of volunteer organizations/Non-profit organizations with Public Service". The council provides an online site for volunteer subscription and additionally provides a guide for all programmes and services and activities for non-profit organizations registered with the council (PSSE, 2015). Furthermore, to encourage the spirit of volunteerism, PSSE has established a very comprehensive web site which includes links to subscribed CSOs and a calendar of CSO activities, as well as access to volunteer bodies in each of the six provinces in Cyprus. PSSE has also created a video clip promoting civil society participation and volunteering at all ages. Even though not broadcast widely on national TV channels, its accessibility on the PSSE web site might be appropriate for younger generations who use online media more widely than traditional social media.

In June 2013 President Nicos Anastasiades created a new government office, the Committee for Volunteer and Non-Governmental Organizations (Γραφείο Επιτρόπου Εθελοντισμού και Μη Κυβερνητικών Οργανώσεων) (Volunteer Commissioner, 2015). This Committee was inspired by the need for more official coordination of the activities of the non-profit organizations in Cyprus. Lack of regulations for financial control, transparency and accreditation, and of a common mechanism to monitor organizational activities for the CSOs functioning on the island, meant that the government could not obtain a comprehensive picture of the volunteer organizations on the island. Therefore, the first goal of the committee was to map the volunteer organizations in Cyprus.

During this mapping assessment, it was reported that there were more than 4800 registered organizations and more than 330 non-profit organizations. The new government committee is responsible for the registration and accreditation of volunteer organizations, as well as establishing regulations for fundraising, especially at a time when there is heightened fundraising activity.

While the Committee for Volunteer and Non-Governmental Organizations does not provide any organizational capacity to CSOs in Cyprus, it has been a strong advocate for the role of solidarity and resilience through volunteerism on the island, primarily through the presence of its acting Commissioner in numerous cultural, educational, and health events. In addition, the Committee has been collaborating with the Ministry of Education in an effort to inform teachers and provide them with the proper educational tools to promote the ideals of volunteerism and active citizenship in schools in Cyprus. Through its presence, the Committee has been able to gain institutional trust and credibility amongst the Greek-Cypriot population. This is becoming more and more evident as private entities make donations to the Committee as a vehicle for channelling them to families in need (Dialogos, 2015).

Together with PSSE, the governmental Committee for Volunteer and Non-Governmental Organizations decided on establishing a computerized management support system, named "Relief". This system will allow organizations to better monitor who receives relief support and ensure more relief equity by preventing possible duplication of benefits. Furthermore, the new Committee wishes to have a help-line available, as well as to build a "volunteer home" in every province to enable people to seek information on volunteering and becoming more actively involved in their communities. The committee is seeking strategic collaborations with Microsoft Cyprus, the Greek Organization of Soccer Prognostics (OPAP), the Cypriot Athletic Association (KOA), the Cyprus Telecommunications Authority (CYTA) and the Electricity Authority of Cyprus (AHK). In addition to these collaborative efforts with the government, private sector efforts continue to support CSOs. For example, in 2015 ESSO Cyprus contributed €100 000 to the Cyprus Red Cross, the Cyprus Anti-Cancer Association and the charity group "Wagon of Love". The private organization OPAP has also produced small video clips promoting volunteerism by showing young individuals helping in the established social groceries with messages like: "We do not close our eyes to what happens around us; do you?", "We can all help", and "Together, we can also win this challenge".

The combined efforts by the different aforementioned institutional bodies have therefore been instrumental in promoting volunteerism and active participation as social resilience mechanisms during the financial crisis and beyond it.

6.4 The labour market and austerity: civil society and resilience

6.4.1 Social Groceries

In 2011 a perceived need in the community of Limassol, one of the six provinces in Cyprus, gave rise to the concept of the "social grocery". In early 2013, following the banking crisis, other municipalities, the church and non-profit organizations followed the trend of establishing social groceries as a temporary societal response to coping with the bank freezes and the inability of a proportion of the population to withdraw money from their bank accounts. Since 2013 social groceries have emerged in all provinces in Cyprus as a predominant example of societal resilience. To be considered for assistance from the social groceries, individuals and families apply for social grocery support in their municipality and, if approved, they receive groceries every two weeks for three months. After this time their case is re-evaluated to determine if they are still eligible for the support. By the end of 2013 there were about 9000 families receiving help from social groceries. That number reached about 14 000 families in 2014, falling to 11 000 families by April 2015, out of the approximately 750 000 Greek-Cypriot population of Cyprus. Combining the number of social groceries organized by the municipalities, the church and other associations, there have been about 48 social groceries in the difference provinces in Cyprus: 15 in Nicosia, 10 in Larnaca, 10 in Limassol, 7 in Famagusta and 6 in Paphos.

Social groceries have been described by the media as a "life raft" for society during the last few years. They offered some hope to individuals and families at a time when they had lost trust and hope in the Cypriot government. Civil society has been quick at responding to societal needs, in contrast to hierarchical state responses that take a long time both to be decided upon and to be implemented. Even though the social groceries have been described as a "life raft", social groceries have also been described as constituting a stigma on the dignity of the Cypriot population. Cypriots have traditionally taken pride in their work and hard labour and many believe that receiving help from social groceries could be negatively impacting the image of self-dignity and self-sufficiency among Greek-Cypriots, contributing to the depression that affected individuals and families as a result of the financial downturn, closing of businesses, and job losses. Some have suggested that beneficiaries be offered duties in the social groceries to justify the help they receive as worked, earned labour. Social groceries have been funded by many donations by corporations which made either financial donations or donations in-kind, depending on the needs of the social grocery. Insurance companies, singers and the private sector have organized fundraising, donating the proceeds of their activities to the social groceries. It is believed that the number of beneficiaries of social groceries will decrease in 2016 as the Cyprus Government further revises and implements the Guaranteed Minimum Income Scheme which was passed into law in 2014 (infoCyprus, 2016a).

6.4.2 NGO activities

In addition to the prominent presence of social groceries, other social initiatives have emerged as a result of the financial crisis. Doctors have been extending their health clinic hours or designating specific hours in their practice to offer services to the population. Furthermore, the church has been organizing soup kitchens, as well as providing breakfast sandwiches to schools for children in families eligible for poverty relief assistance. While hundreds of organizations are registered as Non-Governmental Organizations (NGOs) in Cyprus, very few are widely known to the public as actively engaging in the community alongside the efforts of municipality councils and church activities. These NGOs include charitable organizations ("Cyprus Love Team", "Alkyonides", "Wagon of Love", "Life's Smile", "Reaction Cyprus"), which provide food vouchers and personal hygiene items, and organize fundraising events to support children and families. These NGOs are run by volunteers, with minimal administrative expenses and with funding coming from individuals as well as from private institutions. Even though these charitable associations have been in place since the 1990s, their activity has increased dramatically since 2012.

6.4.3 Patient associations

Major health-related civil society organizations in Cyprus over the years have included numerous patient associations such as the Cyprus Association of Cancer Patients and Friends, the Kidney Patients Association, Association "Life" for leukaemia patients, and Europa Donna Cyprus for breast cancer patients, to name a few. Patient associations vary in their activities, ranging from educational workshops to social trips to advocating for preventive and medical interventions in both the public and private sectors. The two oldest and biggest civil society events in Cyprus include a fundraising walk known as the "Christodoula Walk", organized by the Cyprus Anti-Cancer Society for the last 40 years since 1975. Another big civil society event in Cyprus has been the "Radiomarathon", a fundraising event for children with special needs, held since 1990 and marking its 25th year in 2015. The now-defunct Laiki Bank was the main organizer of the event but the Bank of Cyprus took over the role after 2013. While patient association groups still continue to function as they did prior to the financial crisis, with their annual events, fundraisers and activities, Section 6.5 briefly summarizes the health system in Cyprus and explores how the presence of the Pancyprian Federation of Patients' Association and Friends, an umbrella organization representing all patient groups in the country, has been growing stronger and stronger in advocating for patients' rights and patient participation in decision-making.

6.5 The health system and an emerging champion

We have already mentioned that while patient association groups still continue to function as they did prior to the financial crisis, labour conditions and austerity in Cyprus in the last few years have created an opportunity to advocate for more active citizen participation and have given rise to new and stronger civil society activities both outside and within the health sector.

6.5.1 The health system in Cyprus

Cypriots enjoy good health comparable to other EU countries. Life expectancy at birth in Cyprus is slightly below the EU average at 80 for males and 84 for females, but adult and child mortality rates, as well as breast and cervical cancer rates, are lower than the EU averages. While health status is comparable to the EU average, total health care expenditures in Cyprus are low, accounting for 7.4% of GDP compared to the EU average of 10.62% (WHO, 2014).

The Cypriot health system consists of two parallel and uncoordinated sub-systems: a highly centralized public health system and a separate, under-regulated private health system. The public sub-system is exclusively financed by the state budget, with services provided through a network of public hospitals and health centres controlled by the Ministry of Health (MoH). The private sub-system is financed by patients through out-of-pocket (OOP) payments, with services provided in private practices and accounting for 49.4% of the total national expenditure for health (World Bank, 2014). About 80% of the population is eligible for free care from the public sector, while the remaining 20% of the population must incur the costs determined by public fee schedules set by the MoH for services rendered in the public sector, make OOP payments for services received in the private sector, or seek voluntary health insurance from a private insurance company under group or individual schemes to cover health services in the private sector (Cylus et al., 2013; World Bank, 2014). It is important to highlight that private sector health services costs are higher compared to other EU countries by several multiple factors; for example, lab tests can be up to ten times more expensive than in other EU countries. Non-coordination in the public and private sectors leads to wastage and duplication as well; the average numbers of MRI and CT scanners per 1 million population in the EU are 9.5 and 19.2 respectively, while in Cyprus the figures are 16.5 and 35.5 respectively (HIO, 2012). In 2010, 43.3% of total health care expenditure in Cyprus was government-funded and 49.4% privately funded, with the remaining 7.3% funded by prepaid private health spending, thus accounting for one of Europe's highest proportions of private health care spending by households (WHO, 2014; World Bank, 2014). It is worth noting a parallel trend between health and education in Cyprus: the proportion of households spending on private tutorials at primary education level is above 60% across all income quartiles and is as high as 90% for private tutorials at secondary education level (Andreou, 2012). This parallel between health and education represents the weakness of the state on both welfare fronts: although 100% of the population and 80% of the population are eligible for free access to education and health respectively, a big proportion of citizens choose to pay OOP fees, thus using a big portion of their disposable income to seek private health or education services.

A Eurobarometer survey investigating the quality of services and patient satisfaction in the public health care system reported that about 75%–85% of Cypriot citizens believe they will experience medication-related errors, surgical errors, hospital infections or disease misdiagnosis (Theodorou et al., 2012). In addition to patient concerns about safety, patients experience long waiting times in the public sector. As a result, even patients among the 80% who are eligible to receive free care in the public sector seek services in the private sector, privately financing any health care services sought. In addition to the lack of a primary care or referral system in place that allows patients to seek care wherever they wish, the private sector is based on under-regulated quality standards as well as under-regulated fee-for-service payments. Furthermore, Ministry of Health staff, doctors and nurses have civil servant status; as such, they are traditionally hired and assigned to their posts and promoted largely according to seniority. Health care delivery in public hospitals is financed, governed and administered by the central government and is characterized by a heavy bureaucratic top-down hierarchy and decision-making structure which limits modernization of staff management and the health system in general.

Even though Cypriots comprise a healthy population, the lack of a national health system that ensures universal coverage (UHC) in Cyprus has been a major point of discussion for the government of Cyprus for more than twenty years, since 1992. In response to that discussion, the General Health Insurance System (GHIS/GESY) was originally passed into law by Parliament in 2001. After subsequent stakeholder and political delays, a revised GESY law was passed sixteen years later, on 16 June 2017, and with plans for the new national health system to go into effect in March, 2019. The introduction of the GHIS is thought to be the most important health reform in Cyprus to date. The GHIS reforms include a new system of financing the health care system through the collection of stable contributions from multiple sources, payment reforms for out-patient and in-patient visits, a General Practitioner (GP) gatekeeping system, and enhanced competition between providers and quality-based incentives. It has been suggested that despite the creation of HIO in 2006, the GHIS has not yet been implemented mainly due to cost considerations driven by the global financial crisis as well as by local economic problems, starting in 2008. However, cost has not been the only barrier to implementation. First, catastrophic, chronic illness treatments are covered by the public sector, therefore that patient sub-population does not have a financial incentive to advocate for UHC as it is already receiving medical services as well as medication close to free of charge. Secondly, the public sector in general as well as the leftist, communist party have over the years resisted the idea of competition between public and private providers. Thirdly, while competition is not widely accepted, there is also an overall mistrust in state-run organizations, historically rooted in their lack of quality as well as their inefficiency in service delivery. Fourthly, private providers have never accepted transparency of their services and incomes. Enhanced competition reforms under the GHIS would mean that private providers would be more tightly regulated and transparent. As a result, private providers have been resisting and delaying the implementation of the GHIS. Fifthly, there is a general lack of top-level management, especially over fiscal impact in state-run organizations, to bring about the implementation of the GHIS in the first place, as well as its viability over time. Furthermore, stakeholders other than medical providers, including private clinical labs and pharmaceutical importers, as well as employers and insurance companies, have resisted UHC for their own private interests and financial gains.

The Troika had been supporting the GHIS as a cost-containment element in the Cyprus reforms and the EAP conditionalities put forward since 2013. Agreed-upon MoU health reform recommendations went beyond the GHIS aim to control the growth of health expenditure, including the introduction of effective financial disincentives (co-payments) for using emergency care services in non-urgent situations, introducing financial disincentives to minimize the provision of medically unnecessary laboratory tests and pharmaceuticals, and developing a restructuring plan for public hospitals. Even though the MoU recommendations aimed to control the growth of health expenditure through mild reforms, the ongoing economic crisis since 2012/13 has resulted in decreased demand for private services, while also increasing demand for public services, thus exacerbating the public sector's shortcomings.

Even though beneficial in its different ways, the aforementioned quick response of the Cypriot population towards monetary donations and donations of goods to social groceries and/or NGOs is an oxymoron when compared with the reluctance of the Cypriot population to raise its voice about health system reform over the last 15 years. While the ideal of volunteerism has been strengthened after the financial crisis through many activities of the private and public sectors, the Greek-Cypriot population has traditionally been known to be sensitive to the needs of fellow-citizens and willing to help them by giving donations or purchasing food for donations. As such, to the Cypriot citizen, the response with regards to social groceries and NGO support should therefore not be a big surprise. However, when it comes to issues regarding health, Cypriots have not traditionally responded in the same, or even similar, way; over the last 15 years Cyprus has struggled with a weak, low-quality health system and there have been no uprisings, demonstrations or movements to demand a better health system for their fellow citizens as well as for themselves in case they become beneficiaries of the health system and have to confront its inefficiencies at first hand. It is worth noting that, over the decades, not only have people not come out to protest for health reform but some citizens have even indirectly positioned themselves *against* reform; that is to say that since the employment status of some citizens allowed them benefits in the current system, or they were financially able to pay for private health services, advocating for a change to the status quo has not been an outspoken priority for them. These citizens include the higher paid, unionized employees who are well covered by employer-based insurance, including bank, Electricity Authority of Cyprus (EAC), CYTA and public service employees.

6.5.2 An emerging champion: the Pancyprian Federation of Patients' Associations and Friends

After the financial crisis in Cyprus, along with the prolonged and frustrating delays to health system reform over the last 15 years, the new leadership of the Pancyprian Federation of Patients' Associations and Friends has been instrumental in making several successful steps in advocating for patients' rights and patient participation in decision-making in just a few months – a very short time relative to the 15-year discussions about health system reform in Cyprus.

The Pancyprian Federation of Patients' Associations and Friends (Παγκύπρια Ομοσπονδία Συνδέσμων Πασχόντων και Φίλων; hereafter the Federation) is an umbrella organization currently representing 30 patient association members, the great majority of patient associations and societies in Cyprus. Even though the Federation was established in November 1986, its existence has not been known by the public to the same extent as some of the individual patient associations it represents. During the prosperous decades of the 1980s and 1990s, and in the years prior to the financial crisis, the health system and ministries in Cyprus worked in such a way to accommodate patients' demands on a patient association case-by-case basis – a sticking plaster approach to problem solving. In addition, such decisions on demands and requests were made more easily and not treated with much funding resistance. As such, patient demands were being satisfied, but this was accomplished neither through a systematic process nor through a process that would demand a holistic health system reform for addressing those same demands. As such, and since patients' demands were met in the aforementioned fashion, not much importance was given to the possible role of the Federation as the umbrella organization to represent patient organizations, even though it was in existence since 1986.

However, between 2013 and 2016 the Federation has taken several steps towards changes to reflect the new role that it would like to play in civil society by strengthening patients' voices and rights. The new reality that patient groups and individual patients were experiencing through the financial crisis was severely different from the context they had experienced during the decades prior to the crisis with the lack of governmental fiscal constraints. The decrease in salaries and pensions, combined with the low quality of care in the public sector and the inability to pay out-of-pocket for health services in the private sector, created the need for the Federation to assume a new role as the unified voice of all the patient member associations. Secondly, the financial crisis created constraints for individual patient organizations to receive funding from the government, as well as from public donations, which instead supported the provision of food supplies and goods for families in need. Thirdly, combined with the aforementioned two reasons, the newly strong presence of the Federation resulted from the realization that it was becoming difficult for the government to be dealing with every single patient association and its demands individually; instead, an umbrella organization could be more efficient and effective in representing the rights of patients across disease-specific patient associations. With that vision in mind, the Federation went through a major leadership change in 2013, with Mr Marios Kouloumas taking a leading role as the Federation's President.

Organizationally, the Federation runs on a volunteer basis, with only one recently hired full-time employee but with the vision of two more employees in the near future to support the multiple initiatives and activities of the organization. While a small proportion of funding currently comes from the membership contributions of the 30 member associations, the majority of the funding for the Federation's activities comes from different grants, including grants from the Cyprus Government, the Cyprus Association of Research and Development of Pharmaceutical Companies (Κυπριακή Ένωση Φαρμακευτικών Εταιριών

Έρευνας και Ανάπτυξης; KEFEA) and the European Erasmus Plus programme. In addition, the Federation relies on corporate donations from bakeries, printing offices and venue halls that offer discounted services for Federation events.

In just three years, under the leadership of Mr Kouloumas and the Federation's new Board of Directors and the Executive Committee, the Federation has successfully managed to emerge as the organization to represent the patients' voice in Cyprus. The Federation has gained a leading role in highlighting deficiencies in health care, striving for health and social policies by advocating for patients' rights as well as promoting holistic patient-centred health care through creating synergies between patient organizations and the State. The emerging leading role of the Federation over the past few years has been accomplished through difference mechanisms including the following: media presence and participation; membership of the European Patients' Forum; institutionalization and participation; Health in Other Policies; and creating transparency.

Media presence and participation

Mr Kouloumas, as well as members of the Federation's executive board, have frequently appeared in the media (e.g. on television and radio), thus creating visibility for the Federation and its new leaders and demonstrating their zeal and commitment to be the patients' voice and advocate for patients' rights. In addition, the Federation has also been gaining an online presence through a web site and a Facebook page with announcements relevant to the organization's activities and accomplishments. Building a comprehensive web site is one of the Federation's immediate goals in order to provide better visibility for the organization and for better disseminating information on the Federation's programmes, activities and initiatives.

The Federation's visibility to date has become an instrumental avenue for reporting issues of corruption in doctor practices, complaints about which have increased dramatically in 2015–2016. Furthermore, the Federation has been acting as the middleman body between the State and local professional organizations. For example, the Federation participated in a catalytic role in the conversations between the State and the Pancyprian Association of Nurses (Παγκύπριος Σύνδεσμος Νοσηλευτών; PASYNO) after a major PASYNO strike which lasted for a few weeks in March 2016 and left public hospitals under-staffed. The Federation took a strong stance, asking professionals (nurses in the case of the most recent strike) to stop claiming that they were speaking for and representing the patient body. This had long been the traditional attitude of professional bodies (doctors and nurses alike), who, over the years, have claimed that their demands were in the best interest of patients, irrespective of whether their demands were related to salaries and promotions and not to patient care. The Federation stood firm in the most recent nurses' strike, claiming that patients do have a voice and they do have an organization to represent them and their best interests. To get its message across, the Federation described the strike as "taking patients captive and demanding a ransom to release them". Even though this metaphor was perceived as extreme, it nevertheless offered a shocking image that resonated with reality. Furthermore, following the termination of the strike, the Federation stressed the importance for a common agenda between health professional groups and the Federation, with the goals of patient-centred health care delivery.

European Patients' Forum Membership

Traditionally, there had been a lack of systematic involvement of patients in health decisions in Cyprus. Furthermore, the financial crisis and the negotiations around the agreed-upon MoU did not involve patient groups. As a result of the Federation's determination and need to ensure the representation of patients' interests in Cyprus, the Federation sought support from the European Patients' Forum (EPF). EPF facilitated the development of the first strategic and operational plan for its Cypriot members in 2015, within the framework of the Capacity Building Programme (CBP). CBP aims to enable patient organizations to be more effective in achieving their mission by providing strategic, operational and funding planning support to develop the organizational capacity of participating organizations. Workshops with the Federation's member organizations and leadership provided participants with an opportunity to get to know one another and to discuss the work of the Federation, its vision and its mission. While the Federation prior to 2013 had no action plan and its organizational structure consisted only of a Board of Directors who convened two conferences yearly, membership of EPF enabled the Federation to develop and to put in place a five-year strategic plan (2015–2020), as well as a yearly action plan, with clear goals to be achieved, and actions and activities to be monitored as a way to evaluate the impact of the work of the Federation on Cypriot citizens and patients. The involvement of EPF with the Federation has been instrumental in providing initial financial and technical support. EPF continues to support the Federation beyond the original collaboration with technical expertise, access to documentation related to access to medicines, and patient participation, as well as issuing invitations to conferences ranging in topics from bi-communal patient care to health technology assessment.

Institutionalization and participation

The development of the strategic and operational plan as supported by EPF has contributed to the Federation's ongoing efforts to give patients a stronger voice on decision-making at a national level. The plans have helped the secretariat not only to focus on its priorities but also to strengthen dialogue with institutions such as the Ministry of Health and the Parliament. Furthermore, with assistance from EPF, a significant piece of legislation was prepared, discussed and passed by Parliament in early April 2016. The new legislation institutionalizes the participation of the Federation in Parliament and now considers it as a key partner with whom the State and several institutions must consult for health issues (EPF, 2016). The implemented law is a major milestone and a triumph for the Federation, especially since it was accomplished in a very short time relative to the 15-year discussions about health system reform in Cyprus.

Institutionalizing the Federation's participation in decision-making in Parliament further granted legitimacy for the Federation to be an active participant in ongoing health matters and discussions such as the implementation of GHIS/GESY. As a legitimate health actor, the Federation has also been active in informing and educating patients and Cypriot citizens about the dangers of purchasing medicines, especially generic medicines, from the Turkish-occupied north, as well as online, as both of those options offer lower-price medicines (Koumasta, 2016).

Secondly, in addition to institutionalizing the Federation's participation in decision-making in Parliament, the Federation aims to build an Academy which will be responsible for training patient members from its different patient member associations in different patient- and health-related matters. The ultimate goal of the Academy is to appropriately inform patients, equip them with the right educational tools, and enable their participation in different governmental committees on health. Currently, without having adequately trained patients and patient groups to serve in that aspired role of representation, members of the Federation's Board of Directors and Executive Committee are participating in some of the committees regarding health matters: these include the dialogue regarding the autonomy of hospitals, as well as the dialogue for process reform within pharmaceutical services.

Health in Other Policies

As part of the patient rights movement, the Federation has been in close communication with the Ministry of Labour, Welfare and Social Insurance, as well as the European Union, working together on a new plan that will be funded by both bodies for the employment of patients. The Federation's plan was immediately and fully embraced by the Ministry of Labour, funding has been proposed for a year, and the plan was approved by the Council of Ministers. The goal of this one-year pilot programme is to make employers aware of the benefits that patient employees can offer to the productivity of a company and to the economy as a whole if they are provided with opportunities for equal employment.

Creating Transparency

Prior to the economic crisis and the financial conditions of the past five years, every patient association in Cyprus had traditionally organized its own funding, as well as its own activities. The government has traditionally provided some sponsorship to some patient associations, namely to the Cyprus Association of Cancer Patients and Friends (PASYKAF), the Cyprus League against Rheumatism, the Anti-Cancer Society, and Europa Donna Cyprus. These patient organizations, which also constitute the biggest organizations on the island, were as a result favoured in terms of sponsorship from the government in addition to their larger membership bodies and their larger financial resources resulting from their fundraising activities. This left other, smaller, patient associations unable to sustain themselves financially. The process of granting government sponsorship was never transparent, and therefore one of the activities that the Federation has been involved with has been to create more transparency and fairness in the allocation of sponsorships by the government to patient associations.

The activities and accomplishments of the Federation in the last three years, as well its aspirations going forward, have marked the start of a new era for patient voice and participation in decision-making in Cyprus. While highlighting the remarkable accomplishments of the Federation to date is crucial, it is also worth considering the possible risks that could be faced by the Federation in the future: these could include the Federation's capture and influence by medical professionals, by drug companies, or by political parties, all of which could potentially be strategically using their individual interests in return for funding and support for the long-term viability of the Federation. Given these risks, it will be important for the Federation to maintain its independence from pharmaceutical and political actors and to continue to develop its own organizational and financial capacity for promoting patient voice, and for protecting the best interests of patients against numerous stakeholder interests.

6.6 Conclusion

Positive messages about volunteerism and solidarity, disseminated primarily through online social media, PSSE and the Committee for Volunteer and Non-Governmental Organizations, have been aimed at strengthening resilience and participation in Cypriot society during the financial crisis and beyond it. In the last three years civil society in Cyprus has responded to the financial crisis primarily through the provision of basic goods by NGOs and by setting up social groceries. At the same time the still unresolved health sector reform, increased OOP payments, low quality services and increased co-payments under the Troika Memorandum of Understanding have mobilized existing but low-profile organizations such as the Pancyprian Federation of Patients' Associations and Friends to take a leading role and emerge as a champion in representing the voice of patients in decision-making and policy-making. These activities combined represent clear examples of civil society resilience and hope for the future both within and outside the health sector in Cyprus.

Acknowledgements

We are truly grateful for contributions from our colleagues (in alphabetical order by surname): Camille Bullot (European Patients' Forum), Marios Kouloumas (The Pancyprian Federation of Patients' Associations and Friends), Nicolas Philippou (The Cyprus Association of Cancer Patients and Friends), and Eleni Zimboulaki (The Pancyprian Federation of Patients' Associations and Friends), whose insights and expertise have greatly assisted and improved our research. In addition, we would like to thank the following individuals who have reviewed our work: George Samoutis (St George's University of London/University of Nicosia Medical School), Alecos Stamatis (Chief Executive Officer at the Bank of Cyprus Oncology Centre), Stelios Stylianou (BoD member of the Cyprus Institute of Neurology and Genetics and the Cyprus Muscular Dystrophy Association). However, it should be noted that the content of this chapter should not be perceived as reflecting the views of any of the above individuals or the institutions they represent.

References

Cylus J et al. (2013). Moving forward: Lessons for Cyprus as it implements its health insurance scheme. *Health Policy*, 110:1–5.

Dialogos (2015). Donation from Petrolina to poor families, 22 December 2015. Cyprus, Dialogos Media Group (http://dialogos.com.cy/blog/isfora-e10-000-apo-tin-petrolina-se-apores-ikogenies/#.VtzKSYwrJdg, accessed 15 March 2016).

EPF (2016). Supporting Member's Capacity in Cyprus. Brussels, European Patients' Forum (http://www.eu-patient.eu/News/News/supporting-members-capacity-in-cyprus/, accessed 15 June 2016).

Eurofound (2008). Industrial relations in the public sector – Cyprus. Dublin, Eurofound (https://www.eurofound.europa.eu/observatories/eurwork/comparative-information/national-contributions/cyprus/industrial-relations-in-the-public-sector-cyprus, accessed November 2015).

Eurostat (2016). Newsrelease-EuroIndicators: Euro area unemployment at 9.2%. 31 January 2017. Luxembourg, Eurostat Press Office (http://ec.europa.eu/eurostat/documents/2995521/7844069/3-31012017-CP-EN.pdf/f7a98d76-13bc-4586-9e25-9e206e9b6f02, accessed 15 March 2017).

HIO (2012). Proposal on the implementation of the GHIS. Nicosia, Health Insurance Organization (http://www.hio.org.cy/docs/protasi_efarmoghs_gesy_april2012.pdf, accessed January 2016).

infoCyprus (2016a). Minimum Income Allowance. Cyprus, infoCyprus (http://infocyprus.com/citizen/social-welfare/families-and-children/minimum-income-allowance, accessed 15 June 2016).

infoCyprus (2016b). Social Welfare Services. Cyprus, infoCyprus (http://infocyprus.com/citizen/social-welfare, accessed 15 March 2016).

Koumasta M (2016). Flooding of the market with fake medicines. Cyprus, Dialogos (http://dialogos.com.cy/blog/kataklizoun-tin-agora-ta-plasta-farmaka/#.WUk1siMrKt8, accessed 15 September 2016).

Koutsampelas C (2011). Social Transfers and Income Distribution in Cyprus. *Cyprus Economic Policy Review*, 5(2):35–55 (https://ucy.ac.cy/erc/documents/KOUTSAMPELAS_35-55.pdf).

Ministry of Finance (2013) Ministry of Finance (2013). Memorandum of Understanding on Specific Economic Policy Conditionality (MOU). Cyprus, Ministry of Finance) http://www.mof.gov.cy/mof/mof.nsf/final%20MOUf.pdf, accessed March 15, 2016).

Osborne H, Moulds J (2013). Cyprus bailout deal: at a glance. The Guardian (London), 25 March 2013 (http://www.theguardian.com/business/2013/mar/25/cyprus-bailout-deal-at-a-glance, accessed January 15, 2016).

PSSE (2015). [Web site]. Nicosia, Pancyprian Coordinating Council for Volunteers (http://www.volunteerism-cc.org.cy/Default.aspx, accessed 15 November 2015).

PWC (2014). Tax Facts and Figures, 2014: Cyprus. PricewaterhouseCoopers, Cyprus (http://www.pwc.com.cy/en/publications/assets/tax-facts-figures-jan-2014-en.pdf, accessed 15 March 2016).

Theodorou M et al. (2012). Cyprus: Health system review. Health Systems in Transition, 14(6):1–128.

Traynor I, Moulds J, Elder M (2013). Cyprus bailout deal with EU closes bank and seizes large deposits. The Guardian (London), 25 March 2013 (http://www.theguardian.com/world/2013/mar/25/cyprus-bailout-deal-eu-closes-bank, accessed March 15, 2016).

Volunteer Commissioner (2015). [Web site]Nicosia, Cyprus (http://www.volunteercommissioner.gov.cy/volunteer/volunteer.nsf/index_gr/index_gr?opendocument, accessed January 2016).

WHO (2014). Global Health Expenditure Database: National Health Accounts (NHA) (http://apps.who.int/nha/database/Home/Index/en, accessed 15 June 2016).

World Bank (2014). Analysis of the function and structure of the Ministry of Health of the Republic of Cyprus. Poverty Reduction and Economic Management Unit. Southern Europe Programme. Europe & Central Asian Region. Project Lead: Edgardo Mosqueira.

Case study 3

From Belgium to the world: quality medicines for all!

Maria Martin de Almagro

According to the World Health Organization, up to 25% of the medicines consumed in poor countries are counterfeit or substandard. Despite this fact, there is currently no international mechanism to guarantee the quality of essential medicines sent to developing countries. QUAMED (Quality Medicines for All) is a Belgian research and advocacy platform led by the Institute of Tropical Medicine of Antwerp (ITM) and a group of international NGOs that aims to improve access to quality medicines for poor countries. Its activities mainly consist of raising awareness among key players involved in the pharmaceutical supply system and offering expert advice on medicine quality assurance to governments and donors. The platform is funded by the Belgian federal administration for development aid (DGD) through a long-term partnership between the ITM and the DGD and has for a long time provided advice and reliable data to federal authorities.

The platform's long-term advocacy and research efforts resulted in Belgium being the first country to develop a new strategic policy on quality assurance, intended to be launched in September 2016.* The policy, which is currently being elaborated in closed consultation with QUAMED, will make it compulsory for DGD implementing partners to follow a three-step process in order to ensure that the medicines bought with DGD funds and distributed in developing countries follow high quality standards in production, distribution, and storage. The research and lobbying efforts of QUAMED are also felt at international level. For instance, the 2010 Belgian presidency of the European Union put on the agenda the issue of substandard medicines bought for consumption in developing countries and continues to push for the development of an EU policy on the issue in expert working parties.

Belgium's world leadership in policies on quality medicines for developing countries would not have been possible without QUAMED's cutting-edge scientific expertise combined with its

---

* Interview with Catherine Dujardin, Public Health Expert, Belgian federal administration for development aid, 14 July 2016.

extensive network of NGOs, as well as its close long-term partnership with the Belgian administration.

References

QUAMED (no date). Improving access to quality medicines in humanitarian programs through a network approach. QUAMED (https://www.quamed.org/media/16481/quamed-echo_-_leaflet_en.pdf; last accessed 15 July 2016).

Royaume de Belgique (2016). La Coopération belge au Développement fait un pas de plus pour la qualité des médicaments. Available online: https://diplomatie.belgium.be/fr/newsroom/nouvelles/2016/la_cooperation_belge_au_developpement_fait_un_pas_de_plus_pour_la_qualite; last accessed, 15 July 2016.

Chapter 7

Syrians under Temporary Protection, health services and NGOs in Turkey: the Association for Solidarity with Asylum Seekers and Migrants and the Turkish Medical Association

Saime Ozcurumez, Deniz Yıldırım

Editors' summary

This case study is a about providing health services to Syrian war refugees. Turkey was chosen as a country as it has accepted the largest number of refugees, far larger than other countries, and most of them live outside the camps. This makes it difficult for the government to address their health needs. Of the many civil society organizations helping refugees, the case study focuses on a cause and a CSO representing professionals, the Association for Solidarity with Asylum Seekers and Migrants (ASAM) and the Turkish Medical Association (TMA). This case study demonstrates how ASAM has provided services to refugees focussing on psycho-social support through multi-service centres where it also created child friendly spaces and child and family support centres. TMA has not only provided services through its members but also helped with policy development by providing evidence through writing reports on health, health services and health determinants related to the refugees. The case study demonstrates that the CSOs have accurate local knowledge from their members and clients. They act swiftly and they can make a contribution addressing a humanitarian crisis. The chapter also shows the importance of linking up with international agencies. However, there was still room for improvement with regard to the collaboration between civil society organizations. The authors conclude that despite the exceptional challenge, the Turkish health system has been resilient and that the collaboration with civils society organizations played a critical role in this resilience.

The editors

7.1 Introduction

With the outbreak of civil war in Syria in March 2011, an estimated 11 million Syrians left their homes in order to escape from the turmoil (Syrian Refugees, 2016). As stated by the United Nations High Commissioner for Refugees, almost 5 million Syrians fled to neighbouring countries: Turkey, Lebanon, Jordan and Iraq (UNHCR, 2017). According to statistics from the autumn of 2016 (UNHCR, 2017), Turkey hosts an estimated 3 million Syrians, only 10% of whom live in 26 government-led temporary shelter centres (also known as camps) (IOM, 2017). The rest are spread across the country and have many diverse needs to be satisfied, such as accommodation, education and health care services, placing major pressures on different actors at different levels. Local government, non-government organizations and international organizations became the major partners in the delivery of public services alongside government agencies. Turkey faced a sudden humanitarian crisis and the arrival of a large number of people as a result of its open border policy, but the Turkish authorities are not alone in the field as there are many national and international civil society organizations focusing on refugees' needs in Turkey. This chapter will therefore concentrate on the relationship between policy-makers, service providers and civil society organizations offering health care services (including services offered in order to ameliorate social determinants of health status). In order to elaborate on the nature of collaboration at the time of governance of the crisis, the study focuses on two different types of NGO. The first is the Association for Solidarity with Asylum Seekers and Migrants (ASAM), which is an organization that aims to provide protection services generally to all asylum seekers including Syrians. Services range from psycho-social support with social service personnel to organizing awareness-raising activities. Its operations have expanded in an unprecedented manner in the past five years, along with its human resources and capacity. Its activities extend to collaboration with governmental agencies, including the Ministry of Health, the Ministry of Family and Social Policies, the Disaster and Emergency Management Presidency, and the Directorate General for Migration Management (DGMM). ASAM also collaborates with international organizations such as the United Nations High Commissioner for Refugees (UNHCR), the International Organization for Migration (IOM) and the World Health Organization (WHO), which have been both directly and indirectly involved in the governance of the delivery of health care services. The second organization is the Turkish Medical Association, which is a professional organization for medical doctors in Turkey who have been involved in the health-related challenges of the mass influx in different cities and at different levels since 2011.

7.2 Governance of international protection in Turkey: the legal and institutional framework for NGOs

Turkey signed the 1951 Geneva Convention with a 'geographical limitation'. This 'limitation' notes that those arriving from the west of Turkey seeking international protection will be subject to asylum procedures. As a consequence of this, Syrians who arrived in Turkey as a result of the humanitarian crisis in Syria are under 'temporary protection'. Their rights are regulated by the Regulation on Temporary Protection (RoTP, see the Appendix to this chapter), which has been prepared on the basis of Article 91 of Law no. 6458 on Foreigners and International Protection (LoFIP) of 4 April 2013. The Regulation sets out the principles and procedures for 'foreigners, who were forced to leave their countries and are unable to return to the countries they left and arrived at or crossed [Turkey's] borders in masses to seek urgent and temporary protection and whose international protection requests cannot be taken under individual assessment; to determine proceedings to be carried out related to their reception in Turkey, their stay in Turkey, their rights and obligations and their exits from Turkey; to regulate measures to be taken against mass movements; and the provisions related to the cooperation between national and international organizations...' (RoTP, Art. 1). The Regulation stands out as the most significant legal document in terms of setting the context for how NGOs operate on health services, for two reasons. First, in section five it highlights the primary proceedings for health checks and in section six it lists the health services that Syrians under Temporary Protection (SuTP) will be able to access. Secondly, in section ten it puts forward the regulations concerning the nature of 'cooperation and assistance'. Article 91 of the Law on Foreigners and International Protection also highlights that regulations put forward by the Cabinet will determine all cooperation in terms of governance of the needs to be met due to this mass influx through regulations.

Major governmental authorities assume responsibility for different services including health services. The NGOs and IOs are expected to collaborate with these agencies for all the health care service delivery needs of the Syrians. The Republic of Turkey Prime Ministry Disaster and Emergency Management Presidency (DEMP) is responsible for all the services in temporary accommodation centres (camps). According to DEMP Notice no. 2014/4, the Ministry of Family and Social Policies is responsible for unaccompanied minors and those with special needs. A major facilitator to being able to access all services provided for SuTP is to register with the government and receive SuTP identity cards.

The Ministry of Health has expanded the services related to migrants in general and SuTP in particular via a Circular for amending the Circular on the Head Offices of the Public Health Institution of Turkey which established the Migration Health Services Head Office under the Public Health Institution of Turkey. This Head Office is charged with coordinating all migrant health services. Its services include: contributing to or participating in the migrant health and humanitarian aid activities of the national and international organizations as well as civil society organizations; cooperating with national and international organizations; and coordinating, monitoring and evaluating the activities of those civil society organizations which concentrate on migrant health services. Moreover, the Ministry of Health also announced another Circular in November 2015, no. 9648, entitled, 'The Fundamentals of Health Services to be delivered to those under Temporary Protection' for the governance in particular of health services to be delivered to SuTP (Ministry of Health, 2014). This Circular notes that the Ministry of Health will deliver primary and preventive care, diagnosis and treatment, immunization, environmental health services, women's and reproductive health services, and children's and teenagers' health services, as well as fighting against communicable diseases and epidemics, and fighting tuberculosis (TB). Public Health Services Centres are responsible for delivering these services to those SuTP living in the cities (European Commission, 2016).

In accordance with the framework, civil society organizations are expected to operate in the different fields concerning Temporary Protection, including health services, by cooperating with various governmental agencies at different levels of government. The operations of civil society organizations depend on the permissions granted by the Ministry of Health. The two NGOs selected for this study operate at both national and local levels, and cooperate with most of the actors listed in the RoTP for different projects. Since this study is concerned with access to social determinants of health, data concerning access to food, shelter and cash assistance through the agency of NGOs will also be examined.

7.3 The NGO setting and health services

The main findings of the review of reports for this research indicate that health care service delivery is considerably better in the temporary accommodation centres, where government authorities are predominantly present, than outside the temporary accommodation centres due to multiple obstacles, including an unregistered population and language problems (TMA, 2014). A study by the DEMP highlights that in the temporary accommodation centres 94% of women and 90% of men access health services, in contrast to those who live outside the camps, among whom only 56% of women and 60% of men access health services (AFAD, 2014). Moreover, the social determinants of health (gender, economic status, education levels, working conditions, etc.), culture, traditions, cultural interaction, life conditions (climate, sanitation, accommodation conditions, nutrition, etc.), health services, access to social services, access to education, the presence of social support networks, discrimination, language barriers, the approach of health care providers toward refugees, and the awareness of health care providers about the needs of refugee populations all impact in different ways health service accessibility of those outside the camps, including in Turkey (Karadağ Çaman & Bahar Özvarış, 2010). A limited number of studies in Turkey point to the challenges affecting the health of refugees as problems with accessing proper nutrition and accommodation, unhealthy working conditions, child labour, low wages, gender discrimination, physical and social trauma, social stigma for refugees, language barriers, problems in accessing health services and medicine, lack of awareness about health rights, and lack of awareness among health care service providers about the specific needs of refugees and how to approach them (TMA, 2016).

SuTP have widely differentiated needs for health services on the basis of age, gender, special needs and socio-economic status, among other reasons. Moreover, there is a concentrated population of SuTP in the southeast part of Turkey close to the border regions. The legislation concerning the extent to which the local governments may be involved with NGOs offering assistance to SuTP is ambiguous. Multiple civil society organizations are offering/ready to offer health care services, but there are some restrictions on their operations due to the need for acquisition of permissions from government authorities (IGAM, 2012). Therefore, the NGOs are expected to operate in collaboration mainly with the various Ministries and at local level with the governorates.

NGOs also cooperate with municipalities, especially in the border regions. The nature of this collaboration is varied across different cities. Most NGOs note that there is a major lack of collaboration and cooperation among different CSOs. NGOs assume an intermediary role between state institutions and SuTP for provision of services. However, some of them also provide similar services to those provided by local offices of the Ministries. For example, social services personnel from the Ministry of Family and Social Policies provide psycho-social support services for SuTP, just as ASAM does. However, the need is so immense that providing similar services is almost a necessity. One major problem that has been identified is the difficulty of sustaining services and expanding services to larger numbers of people (MEDAK, 2016). As the presence of SuTP is still perceived as temporary and urgent, the approach of the governmental agencies and NGOs is also mostly oriented towards immediate problem-solving rather than long-term planning and investment in almost all services, including health services. There is, however, a serious shortage of human and financial resources. On the part of the NGOs, the security concerns of the personnel, particularly in the southeast, challenge the continuity and the quality of the services provided, despite local personnel performing to the best of their ability. The formal channel of collaboration among NGOs and local government representatives, including municipalities, is through coordination meetings led by the governors themselves or by the deputy governors. There are informal channels of communication among the NGOs themselves as they operate in different cities. ASAM in particular has been organizing workshops to facilitate cooperation among NGOs and government institutions, as well as IOs. The informal channels also expand through the accumulation of networks by implementing collaborative projects for SuTP.

The literature about the activities realized by CSOs and directed towards refugees, asylum seekers and SuTP currently living in Turkey is very limited due to various data-related challenges. The lack of collaboration among diverse CSOs precludes them from pursuing extensive activities and producing/presenting reports on the activities and challenges at the national level. Most of the health-centred projects presented/offered by NGOs are implemented on a small scale and at a local level. Relatively broader and more detailed reports were written and published by the Turkish Medical Association and the Psychiatric Association of Turkey as a direct consequence of being actively involved in the health care sector. The significant differences in reporting on health care also derive from the difference in access to services for those who live in the temporary accommodation centres compared to those who live in the cities.

There are multiple CSOs, including NGOs, IOs, professional groups, advocacy groups, local associations and communities, involved in health care for SuTP (including those who aim to provide services to support social determinants of health). It is also possible to show that the recent humanitarian crisis paved the way for the founding of new CSOs (both national and international) in Turkey. The UNHCR's last report states that there are many known CSOs working with SuTP in different cities in Turkey (MEDAK, 2016). Another review titled 'Bekleme Odasından Oturma Odasına' ('From the Waiting Room to the Living Room') points to six CSOs providing health care services, including psychosocial support (Kutlu, 2015). CSOs highlight two major problems concerning their role in health services delivery to SuTP: first, it is difficult to track down SuTP and secondly, the CSOs/NGOs have a hard time cooperating among themselves and sharing information. Therefore, this study seeks to analyse the coordination not only among diverse CSOs but also between the CSOs and governmental actors while they attempt to better respond to the health care needs of the target group.

Two NGOs stand out in terms of health service delivery to SuTP. One is the Turkish Medical Association (TMA) and the other is ASAM. TMA is a professional association, which does not receive any financial support from the government, and thus is completely separate from the governance bodies. The main financial source for the association comes from membership fees and professional training and conferences. As a professional association, TMA seeks to promote physicians' interests and benefits vis-à-vis decision-makers and government bodies. As well as upholding the high-quality provision of medical services, TMA also aims to protect and enhance public health conditions and provide high-quality care to the public at affordable prices (TMA, 2017). TMA is noted for regularly writing reports about the health care sector and the well-being of the population, coordinating professional conferences, being active in social movements, and objecting to the privatization of the health care system in Turkey since the 1980s.

As declared on the TMA's web site, 80% of physicians (83 000) are registered to the association, which is also locally present in 65 provinces where more than 100 physicians are attached to each. In addition to office staff (15 people, including four lawyers, a financial consultant, a press adviser and nine technical staff), physicians work on a voluntary basis in commissions and delegations (TMA, 2017). TMA is one of the members of the World Medical Association, as well as being an associate member of the Standing Committee of European Doctors, the European Federation of Medical Specialists and the Association for Medical Education in Europe.

In addition to serving as a regular member of the Turkish Ministry of Health Central Ethics Committee, TMA informs the Grand National Assembly of Turkey during legislation concerning health (inform policy). TMA regularly presents its opinions to the Turkish Ministry of Health and Social Security Institutions, which are the main actors that affect public health care policies. TMA also determines the price of each service provided in the private health care sector.

TMA recently published a report titled 'War, Migration and Health'. This report is one of the most detailed analyses on the state of social determinants of health and health status of SuTP in Turkey, focusing on those living both inside and outside the camps. Though the report does not cover all the cities, it also relies on the reflections of health care personnel who are serving in the different locations where SuTP reside.

ASAM, which has many employees, including social workers, physiologists, lawyers, interpreters, health educators, field workers, and consultants (ASAM, 2016), is a non-profit and non-governmental organization founded in 1995 in Ankara, Turkey. ASAM may also be classified as an advocacy group as it mainly aims at drawing the attention of the governing bodies to the troubles that refugees and asylum seekers encounter in Turkey. ASAM initially focuses on the fulfilment of the needs of asylum seekers and refugees for protection. It also engages in raising awareness and social cohesion activities. It has been organized in 41 provinces and it has 46 active offices throughout Turkey (ASAM, 2016). ASAM also has five Children and Family Support Centres (in cooperation with UNICEF) in different cities; Protection and Psycho-Social Support through 30 field offices (covering 35 provinces in cooperation with UNHCR); Vulnerability Identification Teams in 62 satellite cities (in cooperation with UNHCR); Translation Support Services (in cooperation with the Directorate General for Migration Management (DGMM); and a legal clinic in Ankara. The Children and Family Support Centres aim to address the needs of children and youths, and therefore try to provide services in a safe and peaceful setting. Children and youths have access to psycho-social support in these centres. These centres operate with teams composed of child protection officers, social workers, Syrian volunteers, health educators, nutritionists, social workers and outreach teams.

As a partner of the UNHCR Turkey Office, UNICEF, WHO, UNFPA, IOM, GIZ, IMC, NRC, Handicap International and the British Embassy, ASAM registers non-Syrian asylum seekers (Iraqis, Iranians, Afghans and Somalians) and tracks their case processes accordingly. ASAM helps asylum seekers and refugees in accessing basic services such as health, including psycho-social support and primary health care and education. It is one of the very few associations which ensure psychological support. As an advocacy group, ASAM advocates the implementation of laws and regulations governing the services to be delivered to all refugees and asylum seekers and SuTP. It also participates in policy processes as part of consultative mechanisms for policy-making on refugees. ASAM also organizes conferences, workshops and social activities, such as a movie day with films on refugees, as well as press conferences in order to raise awareness about the conditions of asylum seekers and refugees residing in Turkey. ASAM also regularly interacts with relevant public institutions, IOs and NGOs to better assess the needs of vulnerable groups and work on services to be delivered to them.

7.4 Case studies: reaching out to SuTP for health services

7.4.1 ASAM through Multiple Service Support Centres

ASAM has eight Multi-Service Centres (MSSCs) throughout Turkey. These centres were active for a while even before the Syrian mass influx. Yet, with the recent crisis, MSSCs have been modified in order to respond to the needs of the Syrians. MSSCs mainly focus on ensuring psycho-social support for those who approach these centres. Providing psycho-social support becomes important in an environment where there are very few non-governmental organizations. Looking beyond the temporary stay of Syrians and other refugees residing in Turkey, MSSCs aim to ease the process of social integration for this group by providing services including language courses.

ASAM has conducted multiple projects in collaboration and cooperation with diverse international organizations, some of which directly address the social determinants of health. For example, ASAM carried out the 'Targeted Nutritional and Child Protection Activities for Vulnerable Syrian Refugees in Urban Areas of Turkey' project with the support of UNICEF and in cooperation with the International Medical Corps (IMC) in Istanbul and Gaziantep from July 2014 to August 2015 (SGDD-ASAM, 2016a). This project, which was initially directed towards Syrian children living outside the camps, paved the way for the creation of Child Friendly Spaces (CFSs) either in or near the Multi-Service Support Centres. As part of the project, ASAM also established five Child and Family Support Centres (CFSCs) in five different cities – Gaziantep, Istanbul, Adana, İzmir and Ankara – in order to satisfy the needs of children by approaching children, adolescents and youths in an age-appropriate manner.

For this project, ASAM employed health personnel, such as nutritionists, psychologists, nurses and family consultants, as well as youth workers and volunteers. In this project, ASAM concentrated on the protection of children of asylum-seekers and refugees by providing essential health needs and legal assistance, such as legal counselling and psycho-social support, and mental health and primary health services. Parents are also offered parenting training, psycho-social support, legal assistance and health needs.

The main aim of the Child and Family Support Centres was to help children and their parents access their basic rights and services. To this end, CFSCs provide support courses for school-aged children and life-skills training for out-of-school children, adolescents and youth. Relying on vulnerability criteria, CFSCs' employees have been paying visits to Syrian families in order to better determine and monitor their protection needs. Within the scope of the project, ASAM also distributed relief items and voucher cards based on vulnerability criteria in CFSCs (SGDD-ASAM, 2016a).

MSSCs have been providing services since 2013. The first MSSCs were set up in cooperation with UNHCR in Adana, Gaziantep and Istanbul. Those in Sakarya and Izmir were established in cooperation with the IMC, and the one in Ankara was set up in cooperation with Gesellschaft für Internationale Zusammenarbeit (GIZ). ASAM provides services in cooperation with the IMC and the UNHCR through MSSCs in Istanbul, Sakarya, Gaziantep, Izmir and Adana. MSSCs initially aim to improve the living conditions of SuTP by ensuring health care, mental health services, psycho-social support and legal counselling. MSSCs also provide peacebuilding activities, which aim to bring host communities and SuTP together. Before the MSSCs were established, ASAM staff paid visits to more than 150 families and monitored more than a thousand people relying on Rapid Need Assessments in the above-mentioned cities (SGDD-ASAM, 2013). ASAM states that 129 215 SuTP benefited from services provided by seven MSSCs from January 2014 to May 2015 (SGDD-ASAM, 2013). SuTP are also able to acquire non-food items (NFI) and voucher cards distributed by the MSSCs. The EU has been supporting ASAM in a project titled "Türkiye'deki Uluslararası Koruma Başvurusu Sahipleri için Koruma Mekanizmalarının Güçlendirilmesi" ("Strengthening Protection Mechanisms for those who are under International Protection in Turkey"), at the end of which ASAM will establish nine new MSSCs in Çankırı, Çorum, Denizli, Eskişehir, Konya, Manisa, Mardin, Samsun and Nevşehir.

ASAM also conducted gender-specific activities to contribute to gender equality by reaching out to asylum-seeking and refugee women residing in Nevşehir (SGDD-ASAM, 2016b). Alongside this project, ASAM completed eight projects in collaboration and cooperation with diverse actors including the EU, the British Embassy, IMC, UNICEF, UNHCR, TEGV (Turkish Education Volunteers Foundation) and DEMP. In addition to SuTP, Iraqis were also covered by these projects. ASAM still conducts four different projects – namely the Emergency Response Project in Şanlıurfa, the Protection Programme for Urban Refugees, Psycho-Social Counselling Support for Asylum Seekers and Migrants in the Satellite Cities, and Partner Registration of Newcomers – in collaboration and cooperation with diverse actors, as well as providing services for targeted groups in MSSCs. ASAM has also presented seven new projects: the Migration Network in Europe and Turkey; the Mediterranean Bridge 2015: A Link Between Civil Societies of Turkey and Italy; the Gaziantep Peace and Art Centre; Refwork: Comprehensive Approach to Working with Refugees; the Legal Clinic Project; and Women and Girls' Safe Places.

ASAM in general and the MSSCs in particular seem to contribute most to the health services and improving social determinants of health, mostly through the capabilities that have been developed as a result of long and established presence as well as credibility in the field. The organization identifies the needs for cooperation and coordination with multiple actors in the field and operates accordingly. It also follows the changes in legislation concerning asylum seekers and refugees in general and SuTP in particular and performs in accordance with the requirements of the legal framework. As an organization active in the field, it identifies the needs of SuTP appropriately and fast. Therefore it stands out as an NGO which has consistently enhanced and revised its capacities to serve, through cooperating with the government institutions and municipalities in health service delivery to SuTP.

7.4.2 TMA through drafting health services reports and analysis

As stated above, TMA is one of the most active professional associations in Turkey, which responded to the recent humanitarian crisis through writing reports alongside health service provision. From the very beginning of the crisis, medical doctors have been directly involved in crisis management. Since 2013 TMA has regularly published reports on the conditions under which medical doctors work, on the problems that both health personnel and SuTP encounter in the health sector following the migration crisis, and especially on the health status of Syrians compared to that of nationals. The reports written by the TMA are the most detailed reports on the socio-economic and health conditions under which SuTP live, and are of vital importance in health service delivery to SuTP.

Through its members working in the field, TMA has the opportunity to collect data on the different needs of SuTP in health services. In the early years of the crisis TMA staff paid visits to camps and Turkish cities near the Syrian border where the Syrians first arrived. In a report entitled "Suriyeli Sığınmacılar ve Sağlık Hizmetleri Raporu" ("Syrian Asylum Seekers and Health Services Report"), TMA highlights that there are apparent differences, in terms of accessing health services, between Syrians residing in camps and those living outside camps (TMA, 2014). Those residing in camps are more likely to undergo medical screening as there are medical clinics established within the camps. Syrians are not exposed to obligatory medical screening. Therefore, they are expected to approach medical clinics when they have complaints. As most of them do not have any knowledge about the health system in Turkey, they fall outside it. This is the very reason why TMA states that Syrians who reside outside camps need regular medical screening and to be informed about the Turkish health system in order to access it.

TMA similarly underlines that health personnel working in camps are few in number and therefore need to be supported by further allocation of health service personnel there. At the beginning of the crisis, TMA reported that some medical doctors working in camps resigned due to the strenuous working conditions.[1] Therefore, some others are seconded to work in camps. Yet they highlight the need for sustainable solutions to the camps as well. The report also notes that the majority of health personnel have no experience in working under emergency conditions. Hence health care providers had/have difficulties in responding to the needs of SuTP. The language barrier is one of the major problems that health care providers encounter in the camps. The number of translators is reported as insufficient when compared to the demand. In its report, TMA often highlights the work overload, which prevents the health system from performing properly both inside and outside the camps. TMA states that a lack of standard operating procedures concerning health service delivery to the refugees results in inadequacies in the system. Therefore, service provision does not depend on standard implementation but on the moral compass of the personnel. TMA emphasizes the need for training health care providers on how to function as needs arise in the humanitarian crisis.

In its report entitled "Savaş, Göç ve Sağlık" ("War, Migration and Health"), TMA initially refers to the poor conditions which directly influence the health status of Syrians living outside the camps (TMA, 2016). In this report, TMA members, mostly academics from the Departments of Public Health in diverse universities, underline the importance of applying comprehensive integration policies for Syrians residing in Turkey. Relying on its research, TMA states that Syrians need decent shelter and accommodation and must have access to the labour market, language courses and psycho-social support in order to gain better health status, as well as access to other social and economic needs. TMA is perhaps the most effective non-governmental organization operating at the national level to facilitate access to health services by SuTP. It is actively engaged both in service provision and in conducting consistent needs assessments for both health service providers and SuTP.

---

1 Medical doctors are asked to work up to 240–320 hours per month.

7.5 Conclusions

Despite the existence of multiple NGOs working in the field to meet the international protection needs of SuTP, the scant collaboration among different NGOs is apparent when one observes the field closely. Moreover there is an urgent need to identify the particular health service needs of SuTP and establish comprehensive integration policies that address the social determinants of health needs alongside specific health needs. The humanitarian crisis and the resulting mass influx also led to the surfacing of a major challenge: the need to establish short-, medium- and long-term policy solutions with multiple actors (both governmental and non-governmental) at different levels (local, regional, national, international). There are major challenges with respect to the sustainability of the services due to the absence of systematic reviews of data in the field. The scale of the mass influx, which amounts to differentiated needs of almost three million SuTP and other refugees, would challenge any system immensely. However, the health system in Turkey so far has been resilient in different ways, including having prevented any major epidemics or major difficulties in health service delivery to the whole population, including SuTP. While SuTP are concentrated in cities near the border with Syria, the health services continue to a relatively appropriate degree. Such resilience seems to have been possible as a consequence of collaboration with NGOs in the field. ASAM and TMA, the two organizations examined in this study, point to the different ways in which NGOs play a critical role in health service delivery in humanitarian crises, especially those as protracted and large-scale as the one experienced as a consequence of the Syrian crisis. At the same time, this study highlights the need for further collaboration among different actors (governmental and non-governmental) to address the challenges at multiple levels and from different viewpoints, including – but not limited to – those of health service providers, local populations and SuTP.

Appendix to Chapter 7: The Regulation on Temporary Protection

According to Article 20 of the Regulation on Temporary Protection (RoTP), 'emergency health services will be provided as priority to foreigners who arrived at the referral centres and are determined to have emergency health needs'. Moreover, those 'who are considered to pose a threat to public health shall undergo health checks in accordance with procedures and principles to be determined by the Ministry of Health'. According to Article 27, the 'health services to be provided inside and outside of the temporary accommodation centres' will also be governed by the Ministry of Health. Article 27 of the RoTP details the governing of health services as follows (author's emphasis):

Health services

ARTICLE 27 – (1) The following health services shall be provided or have been provided inside and outside of the temporary accommodation centres under the control and responsibility of the Ministry of Health.

a) Health centres, which would be continuously active to provide health services, may be established. Sufficient numbers of ambulances and health personnel shall be kept available, if there are already existing health centres.

b) Patient contribution fees shall not be collected for primary and emergency health services and any respective treatment and medication.

c) The cost of health services, including second and third step health services, shall not exceed the costs in the Health Budget Law [SUT] determined by the Presidency of the Social Security Institution for beneficiaries of general health insurance.

d) The cost of health services provided, not exceeding the cost in the Health Budget Law [SUT], determined by the Presidency of Social Security Institution for beneficiaries of general health insurance, shall be under the control of the Ministry of Health.

e) Persons benefiting from Temporary Protection cannot directly approach private health institutions, unless imperative emergency conditions occur.

f) All measures shall be taken and necessary vaccinations and scanning activities shall be conducted against the risk of infectious diseases.

g) Competent personnel shall provide information and conduct support activities about reproductive health.

h) Sanitary conditions of personal and collective areas of use shall be controlled and necessary measures shall be taken to amend identified defects and to render the environmental conditions of the temporary accommodation centres appropriate in line with health considerations.

i) Necessary measures, including transfer to a health institution, shall be taken, if drug addiction or psychological problems are detected among foreigners benefiting from Temporary Protection.

j) All measures with respect to the conduct of necessary vaccination for children shall be taken.

(1) The necessary and appropriate physical equipment shall be installed during the construction of accommodation centres and they shall be referred to the Ministry of Health.

(2) Provision of assistance to persons benefiting from Temporary Protection in relation to health services shall be carried out under the coordination of the Ministry of Health.

(3) Persons benefiting from Temporary Protection shall be identified and changes in their addresses shall be passed to the Ministry of Health without delay in order to ensure prompt and continuous provision of vaccination and protective health services.

(4) Foreigners under this Regulation, whose registration proceedings are not completed, shall be provided with health services, based on their identification information, in emergency situations and when they are crossing the border for the first time.

(5) Psycho-social services to be provided for persons benefiting from Temporary Protection shall be carried out [in cooperation] with support-solution partners, which are also specified in the Disaster Intervention Plan of Turkey published by the Ministry of Family and Social Policies in the Official Gazette no. 28871 of 3/1/2014.

(6) If it is mandatory that the health service providers are paid a fee in return for the primary and emergency health services provided under this Article, pricing shall not be implemented in a way exceeding the unit prices or including lower discounts than are determined by the Presidency of the Social Security Institution for beneficiaries of general health insurance. Persons under this Article cannot be provided with health services within the scope of health services costs which are not covered by the Social Security Institution.

As stipulated by section 5 of Article 27, the findings of this research confirm that the NGOs are mainly active in providing psycho-social support services.

Article 46 details the nature of cooperation and support among different actors, as follows (author's emphasis):

Cooperation

ARTICLE 46 – (1) The Ministry may cooperate with national and international institutions and organizations, other countries and civil society organizations regarding the issues laid down in this Regulation and other issues related to Temporary Protection.

(2) The Ministry, upon receiving the opinion of the Ministry of Foreign Affairs, has the authority to conclude protocols, which do not have the effect of an international agreement, regarding the issues laid down by the Law and by this Regulation, with international organizations, within the framework of Law no. 1173 on Performance and Coordination of International Relations dated 5 May 1969.

(3) After receiving the opinion of the relevant public institutions and organizations, the Ministry shall determine procedures and principles regarding the cooperation between public institutions and organizations, which have responsibilities and authority regarding Temporary Protection and national and international organizations and civil society organizations in their own fields of responsibility, in order to ensure the realization or monitoring of rights and duties and the provision of services which are envisaged for the foreigners under this Regulation.

Call for support and provision of assistance

ARTICLE 47 – (1) The Ministry of Foreign Affairs, upon receiving the opinion of relevant public institutions and organizations, may call upon other States and international organizations and civil society organizations for support within the framework of international burden-sharing in order to ensure provision of services to the foreigners under this Regulation.

(2) Assistance and use of in-kind and cash assistance provided under paragraph (1) shall be coordinated by AFAD upon receiving the opinions of the Ministry of Foreign Affairs and the Ministry.

(3) AFAD may directly cooperate with public institutions and organizations and governorates, particularly the Ministry of Family and Social Policies, the Turkish Red Crescent Association, and social assistance and solidarity foundations regarding the use of these in-kind and cash assistances.

References

AFAD (2014). Türkiye'deki Suriyeli Sığınmacılar 2013: Saha Araştırması Sonuçları [Syrian refugees in Turkey 2013: Field Research Results]. Ankara: Republic of Turkey Prime Ministry Disaster and Emergency Management Authority [AFAD].

ASAM (2016). [Web site]. In-House Workshop Presentation on ASAM Activities. Ankara, Association for Solidarity with Asylum Seekers and Migrants (*ASAM*), http://en.sgdd.info, last accessed 19 June 2017.

European Commission (2016). Technical Assistance for a comprehensive needs assessment of short and medium to long term actions as basis for an enhanced EU support to Turkey on the refugee crisis. Needs Assessment Report, 2016. Brussels, European Commission (http://www.academia.edu/28336783, last accessed 6 November 2016).

İGAM (2012). Sivil Toplum Örgütlerinin Türkiye'deki Suriyeli Mülteciler İçin Yaptıkları Çalışmalar İle İlgili Rapor [Civil Society Organizations, and what they did for Syrian refugees in Turkey. Studies and related report]. Ankara, IGAM Asylum and Migration Center (http://www.igamder.org/wp-content/uploads/2012/06/Suriye-STK-Raporu.pdf, last accessed 6 November 2016).

IOM (2017). Migrant Presence Monitoring, Situation Report, July 2016. Geneva, International Organization for Migration (https://data.unhcr.org/syrianrefugees/download.php?id=11697, last accessed 30 October 2016).

Karadağ Çaman Ö, Bahar Özvarış Ş (2010). Uluslararası Göç ve Kadın SağlığI [International Migration and Women's Health]. Sağlık ve Toplum [Health and Society], 20(4):3–13.

Kutlu Z (2015). Bekleme Odasından Oturma Odasına, Suriyeli Mültecilere Yönelik Çalışmalar Yürüten Sivil Toplum Kuruluşlarına Dair Kısa Bir Değerlendirme [From the Waiting Room to the Living Room. A brief assessment on NGOs working for Syrian Refugees]. Istanbul, Anadolu Kultur (http:// http://www.anadolukultur.org/images/UserFiles/Documents/Editor/From_The_Ante_Chamber_to_the_Living_Room.pdf, last accessed on 6 November 2016).

MEDAK (2016). *Türkiye'de Suriyeli Mülteciler İle Çalışan STK'ların İhtiyaçlarının Değerlendirilmesi ve Haritalama Çalışması [Assessing the Needs of NGOs Working with Syrian Refugees in Turkey and Mapping Study]*. Ankara, Medical Rescue Association (MEDAK).

Ministry of Health (2014). Gecici Koruma Altina Alinanlara verilecek Saglik Hizmetlerine Dair Esaslar Hakkinda Yonerge [Fundamentals of health services to be delivered to Syrians under Temporary Protection]. Ankara, Ministry of Health (http://www.saglik.gov.tr/SBSGM/belge/1-44966/gecici-koruma-altina-alinanlara-verilecek-saglik-hizmet-html, last accessed 20 November 2016).

SGDD-ASAM (2013). Multi-Service Support Centers. Ankara, Association for Solidarity with Asylum Seekers and Migrants (*ASAM*) (http://en.sgdd.info/?p=1080, last accessed, 2 January 2017).

SGDD-ASAM (2016a). Targeted Nutritional and Child Protection Activities for Vulnerable Syrian Refuges in Urban Areas of Turkey. Ankara, Association

for Solidarity with Asylum Seekers and Migrants (*ASAM*) (http://sgdd.org.tr/
suriyeli-multeci-cocuklara-yonelik-koruma-ve-beslenme-projesi/#more-1248,
last accessed 1 January 2017).

SGDD-ASAM (2016b). Nevşehir Women's Rights Project. Ankara, Association
for Solidarity with Asylum Seekers and Migrants (*ASAM*) (http://en.sgdd.
info/?p=1100, last accessed 2 January 2017).

SGDD-ASAM (2017). [Web site]. http://en.sgdd.info, last accessed 19 June
2017.

Syrian Refugees (2016). Syrian Refugees in the Middle East and Europe,
A Snapshot of the Crisis. Florence, European University Institute (http://
syrianrefugees.eu/, last accessed 30 October 2016).

TMA (2014). Suriyeli Sığınmacılar ve Sağlık Hizmetleri Raporu Açıklandı
[Syrian Asylum Seekers and Health Services Report Disclosed]. Ankara, Turkish
Medical Association (http://www.ttb.org.tr/index.php/Haberler/hizmet-4315.
html, last accessed 6 November 2016).

TMA (2016). Savaş, Göç ve Sağlık [War, Migration and Health]. Ankara,
Turkish Medical Association.

TMA (2017). About the Turkish Medical Association. Ankara, Turkish
Medical Association (http://www.ttb.org.tr/en/index.php/ttb/ttb-hakkinda>,
last accessed 3 November 2016).

UNHCR (2017). Syria Regional Refugee Response. Geneva, United Nations
High Commissioner for Refugees (http://data.unhcr.org/syrianrefugees/
regional.php?id=224, last accessed 30 October 2016).

Case study 4

Engaging with health research

Mark McCarthy

All policy depends on a sound research base. With competitive funding from the EU's 'Science in Society' research programme, we sought to strengthen the contribution of social groups to public health research through a study called STEPS. Challengingly, we focused on the twelve 'new' (entry in 2005–2007) EU Member States, where there is both less tradition in voluntary and community-based action and less transparency in research policy than in the longer-standing Members. We identified a lead partner for each country, using contacts including university members of the European Public Health Association and community members linked to WHO Healthy Cities. The national partners had four tasks: to identify responsible agencies and networks interested in health research; to prepare position papers; to hold a workshop; and to provide a report.

The workshops reported that EU funding, including the regional funds, was important in widening participants in research and increasing competitive allocation, although some national research agencies found it difficult to identify public health research from within their bio-medical research portfolios, and there was little socio-medical research. Community representatives, recognizing that it was not their role to undertake the research themselves, had a strong interest in contributing to public health research agendas and in using results, although they lacked coordinating structures to have national impact. These findings were backed-up by a smaller study drawing respondents from Europe-wide health representative organizations.

The reports from the national workshops were fed back to national ministries and presented at European-level meetings. Rather significantly, when the relative lack of funding for public health research in the EU's research programme was presented to the Commissioner for Research in person at a Brussels event, and followed-up by telephone calls to the Commission, within two weeks the programme for the following year's call for proposals had been revised to include a new strand in health promotion research. Collaboration between social representatives, academics and officials can impact on public health research policy and practice.

Reference

McCarthy M, Knabe A (2012). Civil society and public health research in the European Union new member states. *Scandinavian Journal of Public Health*, 40:253–259.

Chapter 8
Civil society and the response to the HIV/AIDS epidemic in the Russian Federation

Elizabeth J. King

Editors' summary

This case study is about HIV-prevention in particular risk groups. Russia was chosen as a country example because despite allocating increasing amounts of funding to HIV service provision the response has not been keeping pace with the growing epidemic. The case study focuses on a consortium of health related civil society organizations. The case study demonstrates civil society organization can in principle provide advocacy, mobilization and evidence to improve policy responses. More limited was the opportunity to provide effective services to specific populations that are most in need of HIV services. The chapter demonstrate that the room for effective civil society engagement is limited, if regulatory and legal issues and the financing frameworks are not conducive to civil society collaboration. The chapter also demonstrates how important the autonomy of civil society organizations is, allowing them to maintain evidence provision and advocacy even in a context non-conducive to their cause.

The editors

Civil society has played major roles in addressing the HIV/AIDS epidemic in the Russian Federation, though it is unclear how these roles may continue to look like given changes in recent years. The HIV epidemic in Russia continues to grow at an alarming rate, and affects key populations, especially people who inject drugs. These key affected populations are either not reached by much of the government response and/or are subject to criminalization and stigmatization. The current social, economic and political context in Russia is often criticized for not being conducive to addressing the HIV epidemic. Therefore, the role of civil society in addressing the HIV epidemic in Russia is an important topic for analysis.

The following chapter aims to provide insight into ways in which civil society continues to organize a response to the HIV/AIDS epidemic in Russia despite recent shifts in funding mechanisms and political crackdown on international development aid. The first section gives a brief overview of the epidemiological trends in the HIV/AIDS epidemic in Russia and a description of the responses that have been implemented in the country. The second section highlights some ways in which civil society has participated and/or coordinated efforts to address HIV/AIDS in Russia, and describes current challenges to civil society engagement in the HIV/AIDS response in Russia. Lastly, the third section presents the Russian government's response to addressing the HIV epidemic, and describes its recent attempts to engage civil society in this response.

8.1 The HIV epidemic in Russia

By the end of 2015 there were over 1 million people living with HIV in the Russian Federation (Federal AIDS Centre, 2015). Russia has one of the fastest-growing epidemics in the world and accounted for more than 80% of new HIV cases in Eastern Europe and Central Asia in the past year (UNAIDS, 2016). The HIV epidemic in Russia can be categorized as a concentrated epidemic: i.e. an epidemic that has mainly affected key populations. People who inject drugs have been most burdened by HIV/AIDS and continue to be the population most affected by the epidemic. A systematic review showed greater than 20% HIV prevalence among people who inject drugs in Russia (Jolley et al., 2012). More recent community-based studies have found that 33% of people who inject drugs tested positive for HIV across five Russian cities (UNAIDS, 2016), and 64% of women who inject drugs in St Petersburg tested positive for HIV (Girchenko & King, 2017). Female sex workers have also been affected by the HIV epidemic in the country (Avert, 2016), and women who are involved in both injection drug use and sex work are particularly susceptible to HIV infection (Wirtz et al., 2015). An estimated 6.5% of people who are incarcerated are living with HIV in Russia (Altice et al., 2016). While official statistics are lacking, men who have sex with men are also a key affected population in need of HIV prevention in Russia, yet they remain largely marginalized from services (WHO, 2015).

The response to HIV/AIDS has not been keeping pace with the growing epidemic in Russia. There is a notable lack of government-sponsored public health programmes that effectively target HIV susceptibility among the populations most in need. For example, there is a severe shortage of harm reduction activities in Russia (UNAIDS, 2016), opioid substitution therapy (OST) is illegal (Government of the Russian Federation, 1998), and there are very limited public education campaigns promoting safe sexual practices (Chernykh, 2015). HIV testing rates are direly low among key affected populations, like people who inject drugs (Niccolai et al., 2010). HIV treatment coverage is poor (UNAIDS, 2015a), and linkage to, and retention in, HIV care is problematic in Russia (Wolfe, Carrieri & Shepard, 2010; Pecoraro et al., 2015). People who inject drugs are disproportionately less likely than the general population of people living with HIV to be taking antiretroviral therapy in Russia (WHO, 2013). Stigmatization and discrimination against people living with HIV, people who inject drugs, and sex workers have been shown to be major barriers to accessing services (King et al., 2013; Kelly et al., 2014; Burki, 2015; Kuznetsova et al., 2016). Leading experts in the country have warned that unless new intervention strategies are implemented, the epidemic will only continue to grow (Chernykh, 2015).

The social, political and economic changes in Russia in recent years have had major implications on the response to the rising HIV epidemic. Since the beginning of the HIV epidemic in Russia, the governmental response has focused on screening and treatment. It has not become a government priority and the extent of the problem is debated (Gomez & Harris, 2015). Civil society organizations (CSOs) have been largely responsible for addressing the HIV epidemic among key affected populations (Webster, 2003; Sarang, Stuikyte & Bykov, 2007). These organizations have been funded by international donors, such as the Global Fund to Fight AIDS, Tuberculosis and Malaria ("The Global Fund"). As Russia has made gains in its economic standing and is now classified as a high-income country, it is not eligible for some of the international funding it once received. Also, the Russian government has implemented measures to limit outside donor funding of civil society organizations. In the past couple of years the Russian economy has declined and political ties with the United States and Europe have experienced many tensions, including sanctions on both sides. The economic and political tensions have undoubtedly influenced the relationship between the Russian government and civil society within the country.

8.2 The role of civil society in the HIV/AIDS response: opportunities and challenges

8.2.1 Consortium of Non-governmental Organizations receive Global Fund grants

Civil society took matters into its own hands in seeking funding for HIV/AIDS programming from the Global Fund in 2003. The Russian government did not organize a Country Coordinating Mechanism to apply for funding, so a consortium of five NGOs mobilized together to submit an application and received US$88.7 million in funding for HIV programmes (Webster, 2003). The NGO Open Health Institute (www.ohi.ru) was the primary recipient of the Global Fund grant and has overseen its implementation since the project began in 2004. The project is referred to as GLOBUS (Global Efforts to Fights AIDS in Russia) and its main focus has been on the key affected populations, namely people who inject drugs, sex workers, men who have sex with men, and incarcerated people. In its 2012 application through the Transition Mechanism Funding, the Open Health Institute cited that its consortium would again be applying under the Global Fund's "NGO rule" given that the Russian government still had not focused its HIV-related health services or financing towards work with the key affected populations (Open Health Institute, 2012). Russia is a high-income country and otherwise would no longer be eligible to receive funding from the Global Fund. Since the Russian government is not funding harm reduction activities (such as syringe exchange services and condom distribution), the Global Fund has been funding civil society organizations to carry out this work with key affected populations. The Open Health Institute received a final grant under the "NGO rule" totalling nearly US$11 million for the project entitled "Improving Access to HIV Prevention, Treatment, and Care Services for Key Populations in Russia" for implementation during the period 2015–2017 (Global Fund, 2016). The exception to eligibility for Global Fund grants was made because civil society is responding to the HIV epidemic in critical areas where the Russian government is not, and because there are few other opportunities for civil society's HIV service activities to be funded.

8.2.2 Crackdown on civil society organizations that provide HIV services

A recent challenge for civil society in Russia has been the creation of the list of "foreign agents" by the Russian government in 2012 (Ministry of Justice, 2016). Under this new law, the Ministry of Justice has created a registry of non-commercial organizations that have been identified as "foreign agents"; that is, those non-commercial organizations that are financed by foreign donors and are engaged in political activities. Organizations that have been identified are then required to register as such, or could face a fine. These organizations should then be publicly identified as a "foreign agent", for example on their web sites. For the first few years of this new law it appeared that the area of public health, including HIV/AIDS, was not under the scrutiny of such mandates, at least in part due to the idea that issues of health promotion were not viewed as political activities. However, there is evidence over the course of the past year that HIV/AIDS organizations are in fact at risk of such review and thus at risk of being accused of engaging in "political activity".

The Andrey Rylkov Foundation, which was fined for an administrative offence for not registering as a "foreign agent", was able to successfully have these charges dismissed in September 2016. The Club of Lawyers for NGOs (www. hrrcenter.ru) represented the Foundation, which is the only one of the five HIV-related CSOs that has had charges brought against it for not following the "foreign agents" laws.

Five HIV/AIDS service CSOs have been added to the list of "foreign agents" by the Russian government in the past year. In February 2016 the Omsk-based organization "SIBALT, Center for Health and Social Support" was required to register as a "foreign agent". SIBALT began working in 1996 (then named "Siberian Alternative") and is the largest HIV-related service organization in the Omsk region (www.sibalt.org). The mission of SIBALT is focused on the prevention of HIV, injection drug use and sexually transmitted infections. In April the organization "Sotsium" in the Saratov region received notice that the Russian government had declared it a "foreign agent". Some of the activities cited as reasons for this designation were that the organization was distributing needles and condoms and also conducting survey research among people who inject drugs (Chernykh, 2016a). Sotsium was started in 1998 in the city of Engels as an HIV-prevention organization. In the first week of July 2016 two organizations with main offices in Moscow were added to this list: the non-profit partnership "ESVERO" and the Andrey Rylkov Foundation for Health and Social Justice. ESVERO's work is focused primarily on the provision of services to people who inject drugs and people living with HIV across 33 cities and towns in Russia (www.esvero.ru). This national organization was founded in 2003 by representatives of harm reduction organizations. ESVERO has received funding from the GFATM, AIDS Foundation East West (AFEW), Ford Foundation, Open Society Foundation, International Council of AIDS Organizations (ICASO), and the European Commission. The Andrey Rylkov Foundation has been in existence since 2009 when it began as a grass-roots effort to promote rights-based drug policies (www.rylkov-fond.org). The organization focuses on advocacy, watchdog activities, service provision and capacity building.

Part of the service provision includes harm reduction activities for people who inject drugs and one of the main advocacy activities has focused on advocating for the legalization of OST in Russia. In August 2016 the Kuznetsk-based (Penza region) youth-oriented organization "Panacea" was also added to the list of "foreign agents" and shortly thereafter decided to close (Chernykh, 2016b). It may be too early to tell what factors influence whether an HIV CSO is at risk for being declared a "foreign agent" or not; however, these recent rulings may be indications that it is something CSOs working on HIV-related issues will be forced to face as they develop their mission and plan their activities.

In addition to the list of "foreign agents", the Russian government has also created a list of "undesirable organizations", which are foreign or international organizations whose activities threaten the "fundamentals of the constitutional system, defence, or security" of the country. This law also has implications for civil society's role in addressing the HIV/AIDS epidemic in Russia, given that organizations which have previously provided HIV-related funding to CSOs may be under pressure to stop their activities and their sponsorship of CSOs in Russia. These developments restricting international funding add even more pressure on the ability of CSOs to continue advocating for a rights-based approach to HIV policy and providing services, particularly to vulnerable and marginalized populations.

Aside from these restrictions, there are a host of other threats to CSOs focused on HIV and key affected populations in Russia. This is especially true for CSOs that work with sexual and gender minorities. In 2013 the Russian government signed into federal law No. 135-F3 concerning the "protection of children from information propagating the rejection of traditional family values", more widely referred to in the media and society as the "anti-homosexuality propaganda law". The MSM community in Russia is under-resourced in its fight to address HIV and more resources are needed for the civil society response (Beyrer et al., 2016). Recent legislation has "delegitimized" lesbian, gay, bisexual and transgender (LGBT) populations and restricted CSO activities that serve them, including HIV-prevention services (Wilkinson, 2014). One way in which LGBT organizations have had to deal with this legislation is to add a statement or symbol indicating that their web sites and distribution materials are only for the 18 and over age group. This recent anti-gay legislation has already been demonstrated to have adverse effects on the mental health of men who have sex with men in Russia (Hylton et al., 2017). Civil society is threatened by this legislation, and the longer-term effects on the MSM community's well-being, including susceptibility to HIV, remain to be seen.

8.3 The Russian government's response to HIV and opportunities for engaging with civil society

There are some opportunities for civil society organizations to participate in grant competitions in Russia. Presidential grants offer an opportunity for CSOs to potentially receive Russian domestic funding for HIV-related work (www.grants.oprf.ru/). In 2013 the Russian government-led initiative "Civil Dignity" started awarding presidential grants to non-commercial organizations. For example, the non-profit Partnership "E.V.A." (www.evanetwork.ru) received an eight-month grant in order to implement the project "Peer to Peer" in 2016. Through this grant the organization has been able to continue its rights-based advocacy work and peer-education activities with women affected by HIV, Hepatitis C and tuberculosis throughout five regions in Russia. Another recent opportunity was part of the Fifth Conference on HIV/AIDS in Eastern Europe and Central Asia that was held in Moscow in March 2016. The conference organizers, the Federal Service for Supervision of Consumer Rights Protection and Human Well-Being (*Rospotrebnadzor*) and UNAIDS, provided funding for 10 projects of up to 500 000 Russian roubles, four of which were designated for civil society initiatives (EECAAC, 2016). While these grants offer encouragement that the Russian government is engaging with civil society's response to the HIV epidemic, the opportunities remain limited.

Russian officials, including the Prime Minister, have promised more funding and collaboration with civil society to respond to the epidemic (Medvedev, 2016; EECAAC, 2016; UNAIDS, 2015b). At the regional HIV/AIDS conference last March (www.eecaac2016.org/), one of the tracks was dedicated specifically to "civil society" and there were numerous representatives of civil society in attendance. While there was a notable civil society presence at the conference, it is important to note that some civil society activists boycotted the conference. The following key summary points were made about what needs to be strengthened:

1. active participation in development, implementation, monitoring and evaluation of HIV prevention, treatment and care programmes given the unique understanding of the needs of key affected populations;

2. capacity building for members of key affected populations;

3. collaboration with national, international and other partners in order to improve access to social, medical and legal services for key affected populations; and

4. strengthen the collaboration with mass media outlets to address stigma and discrimination and educate the public about HIV transmission and treatment opportunities (EECAAC, 2016).

Optimistically, these public statements and initiatives may be evidence of opportunities for new intervention strategies to be implemented that take into account the unique Russian social context and engage civil society in this response.

8.3.1 Advocating for change

Dr Pokrovsky, director of the Federal AIDS Centre, has publically stated that Russia needs to change its policies and approaches (e.g. the fact that opioid substitution therapy is illegal in Russia) (Chernykh, 2015). Members of civil society are also advocating these changes. Recently, three Russian activists have submitted applications to the European Court of Human Rights in an attempt to overturn the ban on OST in Russia (Larsson, 2016). The decision to apply to the European Court of Human Rights was made after unsuccessful attempts to receive support from Russian courts. LGBT organizations, such as LaSky (www. lasky.ru) and Parni Plus (https://parniplus.com), continue to engage in HIV prevention and access to HIV treatment services for MSM in Russia. And the LGBT communities (for example, the Russian LGBT Network, http://lgbtnet. org) bravely advocate for protection of their rights and their lives in Russia. CSOs involved in preventing HIV among key affected populations are not only engaging in activism related to promoting HIV preventative behaviours or ensuring the availability of HIV medications, but also advocating for social change in the attitudes and policies towards the communities they represent and for protecting the human rights of these populations.

8.4 Conclusion

The HIV epidemic in Russia continues to expand in the country, and key affected populations remain the most susceptible to HIV infection. While the Russian government has been allocating an increasing amount of funding to HIV service provision, the focus has been primarily on testing and health promotion targeted towards the general population. This has left a large void in the HIV response, for which civil society has taken on the majority of the task of reaching the most vulnerable and at-risk populations. People who inject drugs, sex workers, men who have sex with men, and incarcerated populations are served by these CSOs. It is evident that the role of civil society in Russia's HIV response is crucial to curbing the epidemic. However, civil society faces many challenges and roadblocks to providing these services. This has resulted in a fragile existence for civil society and a noticeable gap in HIV prevention and intervention services for populations most susceptible to HIV in Russia. The most important challenges centre on financial and legal barriers to service provision.

Russian government officials have promised more funding and expressed commitment to working with civil society. While this provides increased opportunities for engagement between the government and civil society, it remains to be seen the extent to which CSOs that provide evidence-based HIV prevention services, such as syringe exchange or condom distribution, will be able to benefit from the newly led Russian government initiatives. In the past, these organizations have needed to rely on international funding mechanisms, which are increasingly limited given the current economic and political climate in Russia. If CSOs are going to carry on in their mission to provide HIV prevention services and protect the rights and health of people affected by HIV, then they are going to have to rely on their flexibility, perseverance in advocacy and legal mobilization both domestically and internationally, and creativity through adverse funding situations. The commitment of the current Russian civil society organizations mobilizing to have a more prominent voice in the HIV/AIDS response and to raise public awareness of the issues offers inspiration for fighting this increasingly uphill battle.

References

Altice FL et al. (2016). The perfect storm: incarceration and the high-risk environment perpetuating transmission of HIV, hepatitis C virus, and tuberculosis in Eastern Europe and Central Asia. *Lancet*, 388(10050):1228–1248. doi: 10.1016/S0140-6736(16)30856-X.

Avert (2016). HIV and AIDS in Eastern Europe and Central Asia (http://www.avert.org/professionals/hiv-around-world/eastern-europe-central-asia, last accessed 1 May 2017).

Beyrer C et al. (2016). The global response to HIV in men who have sex with men. *Lancet*, 388(10040):198–206. doi: 10.1016/S0140-6736(16)30781-4.

Burki T (2015). Stigmatisation undermining Russia's HIV control efforts. *Lancet Infect Dis.*, 15(8):881–882. doi:10.1016/S1473-3099(15)00163-2.

Chernykh A (2015). The speed of AIDS [in Russian]. *Kommersant*, 15 May 2015 (http://kommersant.ru/doc/2725956, last accessed 31 August 2016).

Chernykh A (2016a). The court during an epidemic [in Russian]. *Kommersant*, 4 September 2016 (http://www.kommersant.ru/doc/2967485, last accessed 21 September 2016).

Chernykh A (2016b). The case of syringes. [in Russian]. *Kommersant*, 8 September 2016. http://kommersant.ru/doc/3058883, last accessed 21 September 2016).

EECAAC (2016). Summary Report of the 5th International Eastern Europe and Central Asia AIDS Conference: 23–25 March 2016 [in Russian]. Moscow (http://www.eecaac2016.org/itog.php, last accessed 25 September 2016).

Federal AIDS Centre (2015). Fact Sheet: HIV-Infection in the Russian Federation in 2015 [in Russian]. Moscow, Federal AIDS Centre of the Russian Federation (http://aids-centr.perm.ru/images/4/hiv_in_russia/hiv_in_rf.PDF, last accessed 25 September 2016).

Girchenko P, King EJ (2017). Correlates of double risk of HIV acquisition and transmission among women who inject drugs in St Petersburg, Russia. *AIDS and Behavior;* 21(4):1054–1058. doi: 10.1007/s10461-017-1723-8.

Global Fund (2016). Russian Federation Country Portfolio. Geneva, The Global Fund (http://www.theglobalfund.org/en/portfolio/country/grant/?k=aa469e56-69a4-423f-adf0-ef891eb4a25f&grant=RUS-H-OHI, last accessed September 2016).

Gomez EJ, Harris J (2015). Political repression, civil society and the politics of responding to AIDS in the BRICS nations. *Health Policy Plan*, 31(1):56–66.

Government of the Russian Federation (1998). Governmental Order of the Russian Federation from 30 July 1998, no. 681 "List of approved narcological substances, psychotropic substances, and their precursors under the control of the Russian government (revised version)".

Hylton E et al. (2017). Sexual identity, stigma, and depression: the role of the "anti-gay propaganda law" in mental health among men who have sex with men in Moscow, Russia. *Journal of Urban Health*, epub ahead of print. doi: 10.1007/s11524-017-0133-6.

Jolley E et al. (2012). HIV among people who inject drugs in Central and Eastern Europe and Central Asia: a systematic review with implications for policy. *BMJ Open*, 2(5):e001465. doi: 10.1136/bmjopen-2012-001465.

Kelly J et al. (2014). Stigma reduces and social support increases engagement in medical care among persons with HIV infection in St Petersburg, Russia. *J Int AIDS Soc.*, 4:17(4 Suppl 3):19618. doi:10.7448/ias.17.4.19618.

King EJ et al. (2013). The influence of stigma and discrimination on female sex workers' access to HIV services in St Petersburg, Russia. *AIDS Behavior*, 17(8):2597–2603. doi:10.1007/s10461-013-0447-7.

Kuznetsova AV et al. (2016). Barriers and Facilitators of HIV Care Engagement: Results of a Qualitative Study in St Petersburg, Russia. *AIDS Behavior*, 20(10):2433–43. doi:10.1007/s10461-015-1282-9.

Larsson N (2016). How three drug users took on the might of the Russian state. London, *The Guardian*, 14 September 2016 (https://www.theguardian.com/global-development-professionals-network/2016/sep/14/how-three-drug-users-took-on-the-might-of-the-russian-state?CMP=share_btn_tw, last accessed 26 September 2016).

Medvedev DA (2016). Welcome to Conference Participants of the 5th International Eastern Europe and Central Asia AIDS Conference, 23–25 March 2016 [in Russian]. Moscow.

Ministry of Justice (2016). Information about the registry of NGOs, performing the functions of a foreign agent. Moscow, Ministry of Justice of the Russian Federation (http://unro.minjust.ru/NKOForeignAgent.aspx, last accessed September 2016).

Niccolai LM et al. (2010). High HIV prevalence, suboptimal HIV testing, and low knowledge of HIV-positive serostatus among injection drug users in St Petersburg, Russia. *AIDS Behavior*, 14(4):932–941. doi:10.1007/s10461-008-9469-y.

Open Health Institute (2012). Transitional Funding Mechanism (TFM). Single Country Applicant: Sections 1-2 (GF_PD_001_5efa847d-d50d-4957-95e3-c1263f29848c.pdf, last accessed September 2016).

Pecoraro A et al. (2015). Depression, substance use, viral load, and CD4+ count among patients who continued or left antiretroviral therapy for HIV in St Petersburg, Russian Federation. *AIDS Care*, 27(1):86–92. doi:10.1080/09540121.2014.959464.

Sarang A, Stuikyte R, Bykov R (2007). Implementation of harm reduction in Central and Eastern Europe and Central Asia. *Int J Drug Policy*, 18(2):129–135. doi:10.1016/j.drugpo.2006.11.007.

UNAIDS (2015a). Treatment 2015. Geneva, The Joint United Nations Programme on HIV/AIDS (http://www.unaids.org/sites/default/files/media_asset/JC2484_treatment-2015_en_1.pdf, last accessed September 2016).

UNAIDS (2015b). Prime Minister Calls for Urgent Action to Respond to the Growing AIDS Epidemic in the Russian Federation. Geneva, The Joint United Nations Programme on HIV/AIDS (http://www.unaids.org/en/resources/presscentre/featurestories/2015/october/20151023_russia, last accessed September 2016).

UNAIDS (2016). *Prevention Gap Report*. Geneva, The Joint United Nations Programme on HIV/AIDS (http://www.unaids.org/en/resources/documents/2016/prevention-gap, last accessed 1 May 2017).

Webster P (2003). Global Fund approves grants to fight HIV/AIDS in Russia. *Lancet*, 362(9397):1729. doi:10.1016/S0140-6736(03)14888-X.

WHO (2013). *Global Update on HIV Treatment 2013: Results, Impact and Opportunities*. Geneva, World Health Organization, UNICEF, UNAIDS. doi:ISBN 978 92 4 150573 4.

WHO (2015). Technical Brief: HIV and young men who have sex with men. Geneva, World Health Organization (http://www.unaids.org/sites/default/files/media_asset/2015_young_men_sex_with_men_en.pdf, last accessed 1 May 2017).

Wilkinson C (2014). Putting "traditional values" into practice: the rise and contestation of anti-homopropaganda laws in Russia. *Journal of Human Rights*, 13(3):363–379. doi: 10.1080/14754835.2014.919218.

Wirtz AL et al. (2015). Current and recent drug use intensifies sexual and structural HIV risk outcomes among female sex workers in the Russian Federation. *Int J Drug Policy*, 26(8):755–763. doi:10.1016/j.drugpo.2015.04.017.

Wolfe D, Carrieri MP, Shepard D (2010). Treatment and care for injecting drug users with HIV infection: a review of barriers and ways forward. *Lancet*, 376(9738):355–366. doi:10.1016/S0140-6736(10)60832-X.

Case study 5

Malta Hospice Movement

Natasha Azzopardi Muscat

The Malta Hospice Movement (MHM) was founded in 1989. It cares for over 1000 patients and their families. Hospice services are delivered to patients suffering from cancer and motor neurone disease, as well end of life respiratory, cardiac and renal disease. Services to patients and their families are all provided free of charge. The MHM is a voluntary, 'not-for-profit' organization. It receives around a quarter of its funding from the Department of Health through a specific service agreement. The remainder of the funds are raised by the organization. Patients need help and support to address physical needs as well as psychological, social and spiritual issues. Therefore the services are delivered by a multi-professional team together with the back-up of volunteers. The collaboration model developed by the Department of Health with the MHM has also been applied to collaboration with other NGOs. The fact that the MHM was modelled on an existing service concept in England gave the original founders of the movement clear guidance and assistance in the early stages. Lack of funds to invest in an in-patient facility has been one of the key barriers preventing the movement from expanding its services. This barrier is now set to be overcome through a partnership with the Church, which will invest in the in-patient palliative care facility.

The Malta Hospice Movement provides an important service within the local health system and has retained its identity and ethos over the years. Inspirational and selfless leadership was critical in building the reputation of the organization with decision-makers, health professionals and service users. A high quality of service standards, achieved by ensuring the appropriate balance between professionals and volunteers, as well as the decision that the movement would not seek to duplicate but rather to complement public service provision by filling gaps were critical in ensuring widespread support. The fact that the NGO was not tainted by scandals kept its reputation and integrity intact. This is key to ensure an ongoing stream of small but regular donations from a wide donor pool.

Reference

Hospice Malta (http://hospicemalta.org/, accessed 24 August 2016).

Chapter 9

Social partnership, civil society, and health care

Scott L. Greer, Michelle Falkenbach[1]

Editors' summary

This case study is about running health care systems with the support of civil society organizations. The country chosen for this case study is Austria because of its very strongly developed model of trade unions and employers organizations (economic CSOs) engaging in social partnerships. This chapter demonstrates that social partnerships can contribute to health policy and determinants of health beyond collective bargaining on wages and working conditions. They participate through various mechanisms in policy development and they contribute to the self-regulation of the health system. They have vast influence on workplace security, workplace health, continuing education, wage setting and macro-economic performance. Social partners in Austria contribute to stable cooperation and create a culture of consensus. Despite all the benefits, their ability to adapt to changing times seems a key problem. In the light of liberalization, the context conducive to social partnership is changing. The authors conclude that the success stories of social partnership economies is a testament to what collaboration between a strong civil society and state can achieve.

The editors

This chapter presents some of the most important, responsible, and positive forms of civil society engagement in health policy, namely social partnership. Social partnership, in which employers and unions work together, involves coordinating the collaboration of key interests, freeing the state from deep

1 We would like to thank Mark Vail for his help with this chapter.

involvement in organizing work and wages while overcoming economic distortions and solving collective action problems such as training. As such, it is a powerful mechanism for success, and one that could not work without organized, free, and responsible social partners to negotiate and govern together.

9.1 What is social partnership?[2]

Social partnership at its core can be defined as "stable relations of mutual recognition, institutionalized co-operation and regulated conflict between organized labor, organized business and government" (Streeck & Hassel, 2003). There are a number of key attributes in this definition. It is *stable*: there is an established system that spans sectors and outlasts any single government. It involves *institutionalized cooperation*, meaning that in areas such as wage-setting and training, employers and unions work together to solve collective action problems such as ensuring a sufficient supply of trained workers. It also consists of *regulated conflict*, with specific calendars, forums, and representatives for contesting economic, labour, and other policy decisions, and a hierarchy of kinds of conflict, often with a strike as a last resort. Finally, social partnership is between *organized labour, organized business, and government*. It is not the same as lobbying, where anybody can choose whether to take a stance and compete for influence, or the individual labour market. It is organized into a small number of associations such as trade union confederations or employers' associations that can build up professionalism and trust.

Social partnership, as a general model of economic management that includes health, can often be criticized and has been the subject of many reform projects in recent decades, but when it works it has some salient advantages. It allows countries to control inflation, maintain a relatively egalitarian income distribution, expand into innovative economic sectors by cushioning the costs of those in declining sectors, make stable investments possible, and overcome collective action and trust problems in sharing resources for innovation and training (Greer & Fannion, 2014; Culpepper, 2003; Streeck 1997). It is particularly common in smaller European countries which have no option but to develop strong internal coordination if they are to remain competitive in a world economy dominated by larger countries (Katzenstein, 1985).

The impact of issues such as wages, workplace conditions, and equality on health should be clear. In the case of health care, social partnership works in two ways. One is through the inclusion of the health care system in the

2 There is a longstanding, and large, comparative literature on social partnership, which academics often call neocorporatism. Key works in English include Katzenstein (1985), Streeck & Schmitter (1985), Schmitter (1974), Martin & Swank (2008, 2012), Streeck (1992, 2009), Thelen (2014) and Crouch & Streeck (2006). Much of the debate about social partnership versus more liberal models has been structured by Varieties of Capitalism (Thelen, 2012; Hall & Soskice 2001). The best recent work on the topic, which this account substantially follows, is Hancké (2013).

broader economy, with negotiated wages and prices (and service-sector wage inflation thereby contained). The other, better known to health policy experts, is its imbrication with "Bismarckian" social health insurance systems. In these systems, which often share tightly linked histories with the broader institutions of social partnership (Baldwin, 1992), unions and employers often play a significant role in their governance. There is a sort of elective affinity, explicable by looking at histories, between liberalism or statism and NHS systems, and between social partnership and Bismarckian systems. Even though this role has been diminishing over time, close investigation of how social health insurance funds operate will typically find a significant role for unions in particular (Giaimo, 2016).

Social partnership is at the core of how some countries work, with various combinations of employers' organizations and unions or professional organizations working together to govern large parts of their economy and health system. In countries such as Austria, Germany, and Belgium, the prominent place of unions and employers in governing the economy is indisputable. Even in countries like Sweden, where the scale of social partnership is diminishing, it is still a major part of the way in which the economy and society work. In many of these countries, the institutional structures of social partnership are so deeply entrenched, and the health system and economy so built around them, as to produce a culture of cooperation. Wherever a culture of cooperation exists, there will be some tough institutional or social constraints underpinning it.

Nonetheless, it is inaccurate to say that social partnership is confined to Nordic and Rhenish countries. Certainly, there are countries that came close to establishing social partnership early in the twentieth century and failed, such as the US (Martin & Swank, 2012). There are also countries where recurrent efforts to create closer and more stable business-government cooperation have repeatedly failed, such as the UK (Thelen, 2004). But there are also countries of a marked liberal orientation, such as the Republic of Ireland, or a statist orientation, such as Spain, that adopted elements of social partnership at times of economic stress or when there was agreement on a compelling goal, such as Euro membership (Hancké, 2013). After the end of Communism, the Visegrad countries[3] were able to cushion the costs of transition by establishing a social partnership approach, which also produced the labour peace and strong skills that have made them such close economic partners of Germany and Austria (Bohle & Greskovits, 2012).

Even the EU has some elements of social partnership, in the form of its advisory Economic and Social Committee (ECOSOC) and a separate mechanism by which EU-level peak associations of employers and unions can propose

3 Poland, the Czech Republic, Slovakia, and Hungary.

legislation (Pochet & Degryse, 2016). In health, this produced a directive on the safe handling of "sharps", such as used needles. Social partnership at the EU level is nonetheless very limited. The EU is, fundamentally, a regulatory body (Greer et al., 2014; Greer, 2009). Its tools are legislation and court cases, and to some extent subsidy. As a result, social partnership at the EU level is confined to special access for organized social partners rather than actual government through them of the kind we see in social partnership countries (e.g. there is no EU health system, so there is no scope for unions and employers to run it). The legalism of the European Union and its regulatory focus make it a generally hostile environment for social partnership (Kelemen, 2011). It cannot grow real social partnership of its own and it makes effective social partnership difficult in the Member States.

In other words, social partnership is neither a curiosity confined to a few countries nor a static social structure. It grew alongside social health insurance and has an affinity with it, but elements of social partnership have been created and have succeeded in various ways in different countries.

The prerequisites of social partnership are the subject of much academic comment, but a few stand out. Social partners such as unions and employers' organizations must exist, with strong legal protection. Social partners must be organized, with very little fragmentation. If they are fragmented, then there is incentive for them to seek their own best deal; for example, health sector workers, who are generally shielded from international competition, could seek higher wages than metalworkers who are exposed to international competition. Social partners must have actual tools with which to represent and organize their members. For example, unions must have legal status and resources. Anti-trust law is quite compatible with social partnership, as Germany shows with its strong tradition of both, but it can be misapplied by those who see collusion in industry-wide wage-setting or training schemes. In some cases, most notably pacts designed to prepare countries for Euro membership or to address particularly bad economic crises, social partnership has emerged from a shared sense of crisis, but in general it depends on institutional structures that create powerful social partners in civil society and it gives them a responsibility to work together.

9.2 Social partnership in running health care systems: the case of Austria

Austria is both the heartland of social partnership and social insurance as policy models, and a successful economic performer with an understudied but generally high-quality health care system. This success, whether measured in health care costs, inflation, unemployment or economic growth, is in large part attributable to its strong social partnership, entrenched in institutions and law but manifest in a strong culture of coordination and cooperation.

Austria is a federal, parliamentary, representative democracy made up of nine independent states or "Länder", which are subdivided into administrative regions and then branch down into local authorities (Hofmarcher & Rack, 2001; Mätzke & Stöger, 2015). The federal legislative power is divided between the government and the two chambers of parliament known as the national and federal councils (Hofmarcher & Rack, 2001). One of the most striking characteristics of the Austrian system is its consistent and continuous use of social partnerships to ensure the economic and social stability of the country.

The notion of social partnerships in Austria dates back to the country's first republic in 1918 when the various chambers, discussed in more detail below, were becoming increasingly involved in the political process. It was not until after the Second World War that lessons had been learned to the extent that a repeat of social and economic unrest and discord in the form of strikes and the like was no longer desirable. What emerged out of this fear of discord was the creation of a system, or partnership, that supported constructive social cooperation to help alleviate the widespread poverty, inflation, and unemployment that overshadowed the country during the late 1940s.

By 1957, after a few years of economic growth, the umbrella organization known as the "Parity Commission for Wages and Prices" was founded. The Commission was created on a voluntary basis (Hofmarcher & Rack, 2001). There is no formal organization nor is there a building or budget associated with the social partnership. It was historically grown and cannot be found in the Austrian constitution (Federal Administration Academy, 2014). Simply put, social partnerships exist in Austria as a way of cooperation and interaction between the large representative organizations of professional interests and the government (Delapina, 2008). The system not only deals with industrial relations (i.e. wages, etc.), but also reaches all areas of social and economic policy.

The Federal Chancellor is the head of the Parity Commission and its informal membership composition includes: the Austrian Trade Union Federation, the Chambers of Commerce, Labour and Agriculture, and representatives from the relevant federal ministries that serve on a voluntary basis (Hofmarcher & Rack, 2001; Nowotny, 1993). There are two sides to this partnership: the employee side and the employer side. The Chamber of Labour and the Trade Unions represent the employees while the Chambers of Agriculture and Commerce represent the interests of the employers. The joint commission, as mentioned above, makes up the central level of negotiation between the federal government and the social partner organizations. In other words, there are single peak level organizations representing employers and workers, and they have a structured setting and rules for their conflicts.

Generally, the relations of social partners and their influence on political policy are restricted to collective bargaining tactics surrounding wages and working conditions. In Austria, however, the extent of involvement is much greater. The Trade Union Federation, for example, is the only Austrian organization representing the interests of workers based on voluntary membership. Through its efforts to achieve its various goals, the Trade Union Federation does influence politics. Officially, though, it remains non-partisan. The three Chambers, on the other hand, where membership is compulsory, are self-governing entities that fall under public law. It is the common belief of the social partners that their collaboration in pursuing long-term economic and social policy is beneficial to all. Specifically engrained in this position is the notion that cooperation and coordination are more efficient than open conflicts (Delapina, 2008). Such a culture of cooperation grows when the main players are obliged to cooperate by the system in which they work.

These four large representative organizations, as they are mostly referred to (Gesundheit Österreich GmbH, 2013; Nowotny, 1993; Hofmarcher & Quentin, 2013), are not only interest groups that act as negotiators on wage and price issues or as lobbyists providing services for their members, rather they are institutions that hold a steady seat within Austria's political system.

Their influence within social politics is widespread and diverse, covering everything from their ability to take insight and review legal documents to holding diversified administrative roles that comprise the Austrian social system (Hofmarcher & Quentin, 2013). Within the Austrian social system the partners hold positions within the various commissions, advisory boards and committees of the administrative departments. For example, a social partner can be on the advisory board determining whether pensions should be increased or decreased. When looking at labour, as a further example, collective agreements are negotiated on the employer side by subcommittees of the Federal Economic Chamber and on the employee side by the Trade Union Federation.

Austria has generally been a country that leans more towards the Scandinavian model of labour market centralization. Therefore, it comes as no surprise that it is ranked second only to Sweden as far as market centralization (and with that, labour union density) is concerned (Western, 1997). This high degree of labour market centralization means that wages in almost every sector are coordinated. It also means, therefore, that the peak associations can join together to preserve Austria's international competitiveness by ensuring wage restraint in tradeable sectors (and prevent gaps between wages in tradeable sectors such as manufacturing and non-tradeables such as health care). The Austrian Federation for Trade Unions is the most powerful social partner within the union movements and it uses centralized bargaining to form wages. Of course, works councils at the company level are highly integrated into the trade unions, but a local bargain never offsets a central one (Barth & Zweimüller, 1992).

Four core goals of the social partners in Austria can be identified that display their wide-reaching effect and influence.

9.2.1 Participation in policy-making

In the legislative system, representative organizations can evaluate proposed legislation leading to recommendations for the law-making bodies, naturally in the interest of the social partners. In addition, representatives have the ability to draft texts for legislation that are directly in line with the interests of the social partners (health care, pension, labour laws, etc.).

Because the social partners hold seats in the various commissions, advisory boards and committees, they can influence a broad spectrum of policies. For example, they can leverage the decision-making process in areas such as: the apprenticeship system, inspection of working conditions, issuance of certificates of origin, competition and anti-trust policy, labour market policy and public promotion and funding programmes.

In the justice system, the social partners exercise their influence in that they are able to nominate candidates that act as lay judges or they see to the appointment of justices in the cartel (anti-trust) courts.

The social partners' work in this realm not only promotes acceptance of public policies but also allows for the decision-making process to produce quicker and smoother results (Federal Administration Academy, 2014). Participation in general is conducive to better and more legitimate public policy (Greer, Wismar & Figueras, 2016).

9.2.2 Economic influence

Collective agreements are particularly crucial to the country's economic make-up. These agreements are written contracts between the collectively contracted employees and the employers that determine the working conditions for entire professional groups (bank employees, commercial employees, etc.). Every year approximately 1300 of these collective agreements must be negotiated in addition to the yearly salary negotiations that need to be fixed (Federal

Administration Academy, 2014). The social partners, particularly the Trade Union Federation, can impact these negotiations if they are strong in numbers and are financially and politically powerful enough to back up their demands.

The Advisory Council for Economic and Social Affairs (a subcommittee of the Parity Commission) has the task of providing both the social partners and/or the government with relevant studies on economic and social issues, as well as unanimous recommendations.

A third goal, which also falls under economic interest, is the ability of social partners, specifically the Trade Union Federation, to threaten workers' strikes (Federal Administration Academy, 2014). This tactic is used to enforce the interests of the workers. To be clear, a strike in Austria is a last resort resulting from the inability of employee and employer representatives to come to an agreement on a given issue. In this case, other methods are chosen to bring attention to the given concerns, for example, strikes where workers no longer do their work in protest against certain measures.

9.2.3 Self-management within the social and health care system

Today's health care and social systems often reflect and are strongly influenced not only by underlying norms and values that any given society may have, but also by deeply rooted social and cultural expectations of the resident citizens (Lameire, Joffe & Wiedemann, 1999). The Austrian social insurance system, and subsequently social health insurance, mirrors this view as it is based on the principles of compulsory insurance, solidarity and self-governance and is primarily funded through insurance contributions (Gesundheit Österreich GmbH, 2013).

The Austrian social insurance system contains three separate branches of insurance: health, accident and pension. These are represented within 22 insurance companies belonging to the umbrella organization *Hauptverband* or the "Main Association of Austrian Social Security Institutions". The *Hauptverband* is self-governed, meaning that the State assigns certain administrative tasks to groups of people that have direct interest in them (*Hauptverband*, 2011). The social partners play a crucial role in the social insurance system because they maintain representatives in all of the social insurance institutions, which, as previously mentioned, are organized as self-administrating entities under public law.

These groups of people then select representatives responsible for forming administrative bodies that are in charge of implementing the relevant administrative areas. Those that are covered under social insurance because they are employed are interested in the social insurance scheme because they are both contributors to the system as well as beneficiaries of the system, just as their employers, as contributors, are interested in the system (*Hauptverband*, 2011). Those people who fall into the category of self-employed have an interest in the system both as payers and as beneficiaries of the social insurance system. Thus, the statutory interest groups that have a vested interested in the above-mentioned benefits and contributions have representatives, also known as social partners, located within the administrative bodies of the social insurance agencies in order to ensure that the needs of the people the interest groups support are being met.

In its make-up, the Austrian health care system is an intertwined net of unique and complex actors who find themselves embedded within the federalist political structure of the country (Hofmarcher & Quentin, 2013). It is influenced by an array of actors, most notably the Austrian Parliament, consisting of both the National Council and the Federal Council, the Federal Ministry of Health, the Federal Ministry of Labour, Social Affairs and Consumer Protection, the social security institutions and the advocacy groups (Gesundheit Österreich GmbH, 2013). Advocacy or interest groups in Austria also contain the very relevant and active set of players known as the social partners. As we have seen in the social insurance example, social partners can include employers' and employees' representatives, as well as professional associations. In essence, they constitute the institutionalized cooperation between labour, business, and government, all of which are involved in the economic and social policy make-up of the country (Nowotny, 1993).

The specific involvement of the social partners concerning health care can be seen in the establishment of, and the process of defining, Austrian health targets. This development has been regarded as exemplary at the international level (Federal Health Commission & Austrian Council of Ministers, 2012) because all the relevant political and social partners were actively involved in its creation.

9.3 Social partnership in broader health policy

Social partners (the Economic Chamber, Chamber of Agriculture, Chamber of Labour and the Austrian Trades Union Federation) in Austria have a broad scope of operation in which they use their influence to direct policies and political agendas to support their interests. This section will highlight some distinct areas in the broader realm of health policies and demonstrate how the social partners most recently influenced these sectors.

9.3.1 Workplace security

On 1 July 2016 a new regulation known as the *Zeitkontenmodell* (time account model)was implemented. This is a flexible working time model for the calculation of normal working times making it possible to meet operational order fluctuations primarily in the production sector (Austrian Federal Chamber of Commerce, 2016). As the last revision took place over 15 years ago in 1998 advancing the bandwidth "Erweiterte Bandbreite", this new revision, from the perspective of all stakeholder involved, serves first and foremost to meet the current needs of practice. Given this context, it is the intention of the social partners that both the employees and employers see the advantages provided by the time account model. What it comes down to for the employers is that this regulation will increase their competitiveness, while on the other hand the employees are guaranteed, more so than under the previous regulation, that even if the operating capacity fluctuates, their jobs will be safe (Austrian Federal Chamber of Commerce, 2016). This is a model of employment preservation that works best in economies such as the Austrian economy in which firms and employees, tied together for years, share an interest in preserving an employee's firm-specific skills through downturns (Thelen, 2014).

9.3.2 Workplace health

In Austria workplace health and safety has been a top priority over the last few years. Through the founding of the workplace health promotion known as *Betriebliche Gesundheitsförderung* (BGF), an instrument and regulator has been created that supports the development of healthy businesses and enterprises while providing health support and prevention measures for employees (BGF, 2016). The BGF is a combined effort of the social partners (namely the employer and the employees), the social insurance funds and the Fund for a Healthy Austria to improve the mental and physical health and well-being of people at work. The specific role of the social partners in the BGF network is to emphasize the benefits of workplace health promotion for employees and employers, thus directly facilitating the transfer of these health-promoting ideas into the workforce (BGF, 2016).

9.3.3 Continuing education

In 2007 the social partners created a report focusing on the social partners' contribution to lifelong learning as set forth by the Lisbon strategy (Austrian Social Partnership, 2007). One of the main tasks highlighted within this report was the partners' role in dual vocational training. This dual system of teaching implies that parallel training occurs within a company as well as within a vocational school. In this context, the social partners are responsible for creating framework conditions, continuously improving and modernizing apprenticeship possibilities, developing final examinations, and providing grants and controls ensuring the system's seamless application (Austrian Social Partnership, 2015). This is effectively an institutional complement to the high level of on-the-job training in Austria, which comes about because firms who expect employees to remain with them for a long time have incentives to train them well.

9.3.4 Wage-setting and macroeconomic performance

Finally, the highly centralized Austrian labour market system produces beneficial overall results. Monopoly representation for labour and capital mean that imbalances between rising and falling or tradeable and non-tradeable sectors do not distort the entire economy, as has happened in so much of the Eurozone. Likewise, it prevents Austrian wages rising to uncompetitive levels (and enables an effective national strategy of always undercutting German labour costs by a percentage point or two)(Hancké, 2013). The wage compression that strong unions tend to encourage produces a level of social equality that most research on the topic would suggest is beneficial to public health and social cohesion.

9.4 Conclusions

Social partners are civil society. They show what civil society is capable of when the political and legal institutions create incentives and organizations for stable cooperation and managed conflict, and over time this way of working creates a culture of consensus and problem-solving. The example of Austria shows how well it can work.

Indeed, there is almost no other kind of economy that has succeeded in the Eurozone; without centralized economic governance by social partners, distortions occur within economies as different as Spain and Ireland. In particular, social partnership manages tensions between non-tradeable service sector staff (including health workers), who are less exposed to European competition, and private sector workers in tradeable sectors, who are more exposed. Without it, the result in Eurozone countries has been a gap between increasingly well paid public sector and services workers and increasingly ill-paid manufacturing workers – a gap that is proving difficult to bridge in countries with no tradition of social partnership (trying to force down public sector wages and casualize the labour market is politically difficult and makes it hard to develop skills and quality production)(Hancké, 2013). The liberalization that is supposed to enable flexible integration within the Eurozone is, in light of this pattern, wholly counterproductive. It was liberalized economies, rather than those with strong social partnerships, that suffered in the Eurozone crisis and its aftermath.

Social partnership is not a single unitary package. It is not necessary to import an entire model from Denmark or Austria (were that possible) in order to identify opportunities and policies for beneficial and stable cooperation and governance by organized private actors. This is visible in the way in which countries such as Spain, Italy and Ireland have all mustered strong social partnerships at times of crisis (Hancké, 2013).

There are two main criticisms of social partnership. One is that it is an effective problem-solving mechanism for the social partners but leaves others, such as patients or consumers in general, unrepresented. Those excluded from social partnerships will need representation and some other set of mechanisms to make their preferences known. A second criticism is that it is static, locking "insiders" and "outsiders" into place, but this is an unfounded charge. Most of Europe's strongest and most innovative economies have a large role for social partnership, and ones that liberalize away from social partnership have not seen clear benefits. The insider-outsider dichotomy is far more likely to be found in statist systems (e.g. France and southern Europe, as well as Latin America) that lack the structured conflict and organization of labour and capital. Strongly centralized labour markets and social partnerships ease the transfer of factors of production between rising and declining industries (Katzenstein, 1985) and can enhance international competitiveness by restraining the labour costs of people, including skilled manufacturing workers and elite service sector professionals, who would be very highly paid in more liberal economies (Iversen & Soskice, 2013).

That social partnership is difficult to adapt to changing times is perhaps the key problem. For example, the transition from industry to a service-based economy has been a challenge and led to a worrisome dualization in Germany (with strong social partnership in some sectors and a liberal labour market with high levels of precariousness in others)(Thelen, 2014; Martin & Swank, 2012). In general, de-linking work from social rights challenges social partnership. Likewise, governments have been playing an ever greater role in managing health care despite robust social partnership arrangements in many cases (Giaimo, 2016; Greer & Mätzke, 2015; Ebbinghaus, 2010).

Social partnership has also seemingly been declining or under threat for decades, whether as a result of dramatic political breakdowns (as happened in Sweden in the 1990s) or through slow erosion of nationwide social partnership (as happened in Germany). There are clear tensions within it. Sectors that could have higher wages and profits will always be itching to escape. That category now includes high-salary workers in tradeable services such as finance and design. Tradeable and non-tradeable sectors (e.g. manufacturing and health care respectively) will not feel equally constrained by international competition. Social partnership's viability depends on the balance of forces between capital, labour, and the state, and also on the existence of some external force (such as global markets) that give key players incentives to stick with its mixture of cooperation and conflict.

At a less elite level, social partnership can also become a target of libertarian and populist movements of all sorts. There will be voters and politicians in any country who resent trade unions' standing, view the economy as governed by a cozy cartel of elites, and are willing to support measures that reduce the role of social partnership and unions in particular. In Austria the Freedom Party, on the populist right, has been a consistent opponent of that country's strong unions and their role in social partnership on those grounds (Minkenberg, 2001).

Establishing, maintaining, and adapting social partnership is a tricky collaboration of government and civil society, but the benefits can be tremendous. It is a policy decision, which takes strong unions, strong employers, and a state that can enable them to work productively. As such, it involves institutional change, it is not easy, and it is not the same thing as politely asking unions and employers to promote peace or competitiveness. It is almost the opposite strategy to the conventional wisdom of labour market liberalization. But, as its presence in the world's most successful economies shows, it is a testament to what collaboration between strong civil society and the state can achieve.

References

Austrian Federal Chamber of Commerce (2016). *Das Zeitkontenmodell [The Time Account Model]*. Vienna, Austrian Federal Chamber of Commerce (http://www.fahrzeugindustrie.at/fileadmin/content/Kollektivverträge/Kollektivvertragsabschluss_2015/Zeitkontenmodell_Erläuterungen_01.07.2016_.pdf, last accessed 20 November 2016).

Austrian Social Partnership (2015). *Aufgaben der Sozialpartner [Tasks of the Social Partners]*. The Austrian Social Partnership (http://www.sozialpartner.at/?page_id=2677&lang=en, last accessed 19 November 2016).

Baldwin P (1992). *The Politics of Social Solidarity: Class Bases of the European Welfare State, 1975–1975*. Cambridge, Cambridge University Press.

Barth E, Zweimüller J (1992). Labour market institutions and the industry wage distribution – Evidence from Austria, Norway and the US. *Empirica*, 19(2):181–201. doi.org/10.1007/BF00924960.

BGF (2016). *Erfolgsfaktor Gesundheit am Arbeitsplatz [Health Success Factor in the Workplace]*. Linz, Betriebliche Gesundheitsförderung (http://www.netzwerk-bgf.at/cdscontent/load?contentid=10008.631183&version=1464856031, last accessed 20 November 2016).

Bohle D, Greskovits B (2012). *Capitalist Diversity on Europe's Periphery*. Ithaca, Cornell University Press.

CEP (2014). *Gesundheit und Sicherheit am Arbeitsplatz [Health and Safety at Work]*. Centre for European Politics (http://www.cep.eu/Analysen/COM_2014_332_Gesundheit_und_Sicherheit/cepAnalyse_COM_2014_332_Gesundheit_und_Sicherheit_am_Arbeitsplatz.pdf, last accessed 20 November 2016).

Crouch C, Streeck W (2006). *The diversity of democracy: corporatism, social order and political conflict*. Cheltenham, Edward Elgar Publishing.

Culpepper PD (2003). *Creating Cooperation: How States Develop Human Capital in Europe*. Ithaca, Cornell University Press.

Delapina T (2008). *The Austrian Social Partnership*. Brussels.

Ebbinghaus B (2010). Reforming Bismarckian corporatism: The changing role of social partnership in continental Europe. In Palier B, ed., *A long goodbye to Bismarck? The Politics of Welfare Reform in Continental Europe*. Amsterdam, Amsterdam University Press, 255–278.

Federal Administration Academy (2014). *Sozialpartner [Social Partners]*. Vienna, Federal Administration Academy (https://www.oeffentlicherdienst.gv.at/vab/seminarprogramm/allgemeine_ausbildung_und_weiterbildung/Kapitel_10_Sozialpartner.pdf?5i7woz, last accessed 19 November 2016).

Federal Health Commission & Austrian Council of Ministers (2012). Health In All Policies – Health Targets Austria. Federal Health Commission & Austrian Council of Ministers (http://www.gesundheitsziele-oesterreich.at/austrian-health-targets/, last accessed 13 November 2016).

Gesundheit Österreich GmbH (2013). *Das Österreichische Gesundheitssystem-Zahlen-Daten-Fakten [The Austrian Health System: Facts and Figures]*. Vienna, Gesundheit Österreich GmbH.

Giaimo S (2016). *Reforming Health Care in the United States, Germany, and South Africa: Comparative Perspectives on Health*. New York, Palgrave Macmillan US.

Greer SL (2009). Ever Closer Union: Devolution, the European Union, and Social Citizenship Rights. In Greer SL, ed., *Devolution and Social Citizenship Rights in the United Kingdom*. Bristol, Policy, 175–196.

Greer SL, Fannion RD (2014). I'll Be Gone, You'll Be Gone: Why American Employers Underinvest in Health. *Journal of health politics, policy and law*, 39(5):989–1012.

Greer SL, Mätzke M (2015). Health Policy in the European Union. In Kuhlmann E et al., eds., *The Palgrave International Handbook of Healthcare Policy and Governance*. Basingstoke. Palgrave Macmillan.

Greer SL, Wismar M, Figueras J, eds. (2016). *Strengthening health system governance: better policies, stronger performance*. Maidenhead, Open University Press.

Greer SL et al. (2014). *Everything you always wanted to know about European Union health policy but were afraid to ask*. Copenhagen, WHO Regional Office for Europe on behalf of the European Observatory on Health Systems and Policies.

Hall PA, Soskice D (2001). *Varieties of Capitalism: The Institutional Foundations of Comparative Advantage*. Oxford, Oxford University Press.

Hancké B (2013). *Unions, Central Banks, and EMU: Labour Market Institutions and Monetary Integration in Europe*. Oxford, Oxford University Press.

Hauptverband (2011). *Die Organisation der österreichischen Sozialversicherung Selbstverwaltung [Main Association of Austrian Social Security Institutions]*. Vienna, Hauptverband (http://www.hauptverband.at/cdscontent/load?conten tid=10008.564266&version=1391184549, last accessed 13 November 2016).

Hofmarcher MM, Quentin W (2013). *Das österreichische Gesundheitssystem: Akteure, Daten, Analysen*. Berlin, Medizinisch Wissenschaftliche Verlagsgesellschaft.

Hofmarcher MM, Rack H (2001). *Health care systems in transition: Austria*. Copenhagen, European Observatory on Health Care Systems.

Iversen T, Soskice D (2013). A political-institutional model of real exchange rates, competitiveness, and the division of labor. In Wren A, ed., *The Political Economy of the Service Transition*. Oxford, Oxford University Press, 73–107.

Katzenstein PJ (1985). *Small States in World Markets: Industrial Policy in Europe*. Ithaca, Cornell University Press.

Kelemen RD (2011). *Eurolegalism: The Transformation of Law and Regulation in the European Union*. Cambridge, MA, Harvard University Press.

Lameire N, Joffe P, Wiedemann M (1999). Healthcare systems – an international review: an overview. *Nephrology Dialysis Transplantation*, 14(suppl 6):3–9. doi. org/10.1093/ndt/14.suppl_6.3.

Martin CJ, Swank D (2008). The Political Origins of Coordinated Capitalism: Business Organizations, Party Systems, and State Structure in the Age of Innocence. *American Political Science Review*, 102(2):181–198.

Martin CJ, Swank D (2012). *The political construction of business interests: coordination, growth, and equality*. Cambridge, Cambridge University Press.

Mätzke M, Stöger H (2015). Austria. In Fierlbeck K, Palley HA, eds., *Comparative Health Care Federalism*. Farnham, Ashgate, 15–29.

Minkenberg M (2001). The radical right in public office: Agenda-setting and policy effects. *West European Politics*, 24(4):1–21.

Nowotny E (1993). The Austrian Social Partnership and Democracy. Minneapolis, MN, University of Minnesota, Center for Austrian Studies, Working Paper 93-1.

Pochet P, Degryse C (2016). *Dialogue social européen: une relance «de la dernière chance»?* Brussels, European Social Observatory, Opinion Paper no. 17.

Schmitter PC (1974). Still the Century of Corporatism? *The Review of Politics*, 36:85–131.

Streeck W (1992). Productive Constraints: on the Institutional Conditions of Diversified Quality Production. In Streeck W, ed., *Social Institutions and Economic Performance: Industrial Relations in Advanced Capitalist Countries*. Newbury Park, CA, Sage, 1–40.

Streeck W (1997). Beneficial constraints: on the economic limits of rational voluntarism. In Rogers Hollingsworth J, Boyer R, eds., *Contemporary capitalism: The embeddedness of institutions*. Cambridge, Cambridge University Press, 197–219.

Streeck W (2009). *Re-forming capitalism: Institutional change in the German political economy*. Oxford, Oxford University Press on Demand.

Streeck W, Hassel A (2003). The crumbling pillars of social partnership. *West European Politics*, 26(4):101–124.

Streeck W, Schmitter PC (1985). Community, market, state – and associations? The prospective contribution of interest governance to social order. In Streeck W, Schmitter PC, eds., *Private Interest Government: Beyond Market and State*. London, Sage, 1–29.

Thelen K (2004). *How Institutions Evolve: The Political Economy of Skills in Germany, Britain, the United States, and Japan.* Cambridge, Cambridge University Press.

Thelen K (2012). Varieties of capitalism: Trajectories of liberalization and the new politics of social solidarity. *Annual Review of Political Science*, 15:137–159.

Thelen K (2014). *Varieties of liberalization and the new politics of social solidarity.* Cambridge, Cambridge University Press.

Western B (1997). *Between Class and Market: Postwar Unionization in the Capitalist Democracies.* Princeton, Princeton University Press.

Case study 6

Civil Society and the Refugee Crisis in Germany 2015/16

Andreas Schmid, Molly Green

In 2015 Germany experienced a huge influx of refugees as more than 850 000 people crossed the border, mainly in the southern part of Bavaria. Over 40 000 of them were unaccompanied children[1]. On many days, thousands walked into this rural part of Germany with no place to go and little idea of what to expect.

Two stages followed the arrival; the first stage involved short-term logistics of processing refugees, and the second (ongoing) stage involves long-term efforts with the refugee population.

During the first stage there was an outstanding societal response which, especially in the arrival hotspots, translated into unconditional help: setting up shelters, running soup kitchens, collecting and distributing clothing, etc. From firefighters to Catholic youth groups, local Red Cross chapters or volunteers without affiliation, people lent a helping hand. These informal structures and responses were quick and compassionate, and filled many gaps in the response from government agencies. This continued as the first waves of refugees were distributed across Germany[2].

The responsibility for the second stage lies primarily with the counties, resulting in heterogeneous strategies and outcomes. Many local governments have been overwhelmed by the tasks of refugee settlement and integration. Refugees often compete with local residents for resources, including affordable housing, and the federal government policy often didn't extend well to the local level[3].

The extensive engagement of civil society in the first months has subsequently decreased, as many volunteers have tired of the high workload and are frustrated by a lack of perspective. One main cause is a change in politics, including an acknowledgment that full integration of all the refugees will not be possible and many will have to return home. Many volunteers feel this counteracts all the efforts that they have made to facilitate integration of these individuals[4,5].

The second stage is, and will continue to be, a huge challenge. A coherent long-term strategy is still in the making, and very controversial debates as to whether the (mostly muslim) refugees are compatible with German culture and with the continued peace and safety of Germany and its citizens are gaining momentum (Funk, 2016).

References

[1] Hillmann L, Dufner A (In press). Refugee Children in Germany. *Journal of Ethnic and Migration Studies.*

[2] Funk N (2016). A spectre in Germany: refugees, a 'welcome culture' and 'integration politics'. *Journal of Global Ethics*, 12(3):289–299.

[3] Laubenthal B (2016). Political institutions and asylum policies – the case of Germany. *Psychosociological Issues in Human Resource Management*, 4(2):122–144.

[4] Wirth G (2017). Abschiebung während der Lehre [Deportation during teaching]. http://www.br.de/nachrichten/fluechtlinge-abschiebung-integration-100.html, accessed 12 February 2017.

[5] Trauner F (2016). Asylum policy: the EU's 'crises' and the looming policy regime failure. *Journal of European Integration*, 38(3):311–325. DOI:10.1080/07036337.2016.1140756.

Chapter 10

The conditions and contributions of 'Whole of Society' governance in the Dutch 'All about Health...' programme

Marleen Bekker, Jan Kees Helderman, Maria Jansen, Dirk Ruwaard
Funding: This work was supported by the Netherlands Organization for
Health Research and Development (ZonMw) [grant no. 531005010]

Editors' summary

This chapter is about a programme called "All about Health..." the
programme aims at improving health by engaging all members of society
in a social health movement, which greatly resembles a whole-of-society
approach. The country chosen for this case study is the Netherlands, as the
government and numerous organizations have engaged in collaboration.
There are various CSOs, commercial partners, municipalities and
government agencies and services involved. While there are many concrete
health related "pledges" made between the partners of the programme,
the overall aim is to move from government to governance and to involve
many more stakeholders in policy making and implementation at all
levels. Most prominently, partners organised events and provided services
to the public. Additionally, they provided evidence, contributed to policy
developed, exercised advocacy, helped consensus building, acted as watch
dogs, provided services and acted as self-regulators. Strong government
support, a small programme office and an ongoing programme evaluation
have been instrumental to the progress of the programme. The authors
conclude that the first three years of "All about Health..." seems to provide

an early backing of the hypotheses that CSOs contribute to health though it is too early for a final assessment.

The editors

10.1 Introduction

This chapter will describe and analyse a particular example of a governmental programme enhancing collaborative public, private and CSO initiatives for health: "All about Health…" (2014–2016). Interestingly, in this programme the Dutch government recognizes the potential these organizations have to offer in increasing the reach, acceptance and impact of targeted groups. Early experiences in this programme can help us to analyse conditions and challenges for sustained CSO initiative and their early contributions. In 2015 and 2016 Maastricht University and Radboud University conducted a qualitative monitoring study into the governance aspects of this programme. In this chapter we will address the following questions:

1. Which **activities** do CSO partners of the "All about Health…" programme contribute?

2. How do governments and CSOs develop **dialogue and collaboration** in practice?

3. Which **conditions** emerge for developing further the "All about Health…" programme as a 'whole of society' approach, and for achieving its health goals and ambitions?

Before we address these questions, we start with a contextual exploration of historical trends and current challenges in Dutch state-society relationships to understand how these may or may not shape or contribute to the role of CSOs in public health in the Netherlands. This section ends with a description of the current challenges in public health with regard to the potential role of CSOs. The third section is devoted to the general framework, research methods and findings of the "All about Health…" programme. In this section the three questions above will be answered.[1] We end with conclusions about the move from government to health governance, and the conditions for engaging with CSOs.

10.2 State-society relations and public health challenges in the Netherlands

In this section we investigate the relationships between the state and organized

---

1 Parts of this analysis were discussed during workshops with the European Observatory on Health Systems and Policies and the WHO Office for Europe at the EPH conferences in 2015 (Milan) and 2016 (Vienna).

civil society, between the state and the market, and between the state and the community, ending with the specific public health challenges.

10.2.1 Trends in the relationship between the state and organized civil society

The Netherlands is a decentralized unitary state. It has a long-standing tradition of well organized CSOs sharing responsibility with the state for policy-making and service delivery in a wide variety of policy domains, such as open water management, spatial planning and social services (Hemerijck, 1992; Brandsen & Pape, 2015). The Dutch private health care system, for example, has been built upon *corporatist arrangements*, whereby the state shares its public regulatory authority with the various associations of providers, insurers, trade unions and employers (Helderman, 2007). The *public health sector*, however, has never been part of these well established corporatist institutions and practices in the Netherlands. Article 22 of the Dutch Constitution stipulates that the government shall take measures "for the promotion of the health of the public", but it led to two discrete and only loosely coupled policy circuits (Bekker & Putters, 2003). In the post-war era of welfare state expansion, the Dutch health care system became, on the one hand, a classic example of a corporatist social health insurance system with predominantly public financing and a private delivery of health care (Helderman et al., 2005). Public health, on the other hand, had largely been delegated to the local municipalities. In the Dutch decentralized unitary state, municipalities were obliged to establish and maintain Municipal Health Services to perform these tasks.

As a consequence, health policies in the Netherlands used to be dominated by the technical and financial details of the health insurance system and the curative health care and medical sector, at the cost of the broader issue of public health promotion and prevention (Mackenbach, 2003). Meanwhile, public health consisted of a mostly *unilateral, state-dictated* policy and framework for local services. Since the general belief for a long time has been that there would be no "public demand" for prevention, standardized expert tasks in public health developed at a distance from both the citizens and CSOs.

But even if public health policies could theoretically have benefited from experiences with the Dutch corporatist mode of collaborative governance, *corporatism itself has eroded* under the influence of neoliberal governance in the 1980s and 1990s and the financial-economic crisis (2007–2012) (Brandsen & Pape, 2015). For about 80 years Dutch coalition cabinets were dominated by the Christian-Democrats, effectively deploying consensual policy-making with representatives of majority and minority interests. Under the historic "Purple cabinet" (1994–2002), however, the socio-liberal government decided that policies should become more evidence-based rather than interest-based. In the second half of the 1990s corporatist intermediary associations evolved into branch organizations, while the former corporatist Advisory Councils were converted into science-based knowledge institutes or independent regulatory agencies (Putters & Twist, 2007; Bekker et al. 2010; Helderman, Bevan & France, 2012).

10.2.2 Trends in the relationship between the state and the market

While these formerly corporatist associations try to strike a new balance between being a branch service organization and an effective representative interest organization, successive governments have started experimenting with new kinds of *"collaborative governance"*, mobilizing civil society and corporate sources for public problem-solving. Going beyond more traditional subsidy programmes and social insurance schemes, government in several policy areas developed covenants, public-private partnerships and "Deals" directly with community and commercial entrepreneurs. Gradually, the role of government is changing towards facilitating an independent committee or long-term commissioner, who designs a general framework of requirements or guidelines, and monitors progress. The government positions itself as a more equal, relatively neutral, and facilitative partner. Examples are the Green Deals programme (Van Mil et al., 2013) or the Delta commissioner,[2] who has recently been appointed by the government to a second term of seven years (Jong & Brink, 2013).

In commercial industries there is also a growing awareness of *corporate social responsibility* (Carroll, 1991). Publicity concerning incidental or structural risks and wrongs of corporate activities with regard to environment and health in the past decade have resulted in consumer power and boycotts, and corporate management of externalities beyond business damage control. An eight-year governmental programme on Corporate Social Responsibility developed corporate support and CSO expertise (MVO Nederland, 2013). More than 2000 corporate partners now pay a membership fee to the independent CSR Netherlands foundation[3] developing corporate norms, and offering CSR expertise and change management services. CSR awareness is now moving beyond managing externalities towards incorporation into the operational core of business organizations. Even though at this stage this is an "early adopter" practice, it is exemplary of proactive efforts integrating "social capital policies" into economic business plans, such as sustainable labour participation, healthy production chains, or advanced consumer feedback methods, regional stakeholder dialogues and co-production chains. At the same time, *health in itself has become a marketed product and service*, focusing primarily on lifestyle

---

2 See for more info respectively, http://www.greendeals.nl/english and https://english.deltacommissaris.nl/.

3 For more info see http://mvonederland.nl/csr-netherlands.

coaching, food, physical and social activity services as well as medical(-ized) products in medicines, medical aids, e-health apps and web tools, and other products for self-diagnosis and self-treatment.

10.2.3 Trends in the role of the state and the community

As a consequence of the highly institutionalized corporatist nature of the Dutch welfare state, with its reliance on social insurance schemes, citizens' initiatives and community involvement in social welfare provision have been rather limited in the Netherlands. But in the last decade, in response to reforms of the financially unsustainable social security system and the long-term care system, successive governments stress the *need for more self-reliance, autonomy and informal care* among citizens and community groups. In his first Annual Speech to Parliament in 2013, King William-Alexander spoke about the need to revitalize communitarian involvement and citizens' participation in the welfare state (National Government of the Netherlands, 2013). With welfare state retrenchment and reforms, the rising share in GDP of health care expenditures and other welfare support costs, and the financial crisis, government now turns its public call for more citizen and community responsibility into *legal and financial measures*. For instance, in the Youth Act the former citizen's "right to care or assistance" is now replaced with a state obligation to provide support "when necessary" with regards to the family supportive capacity (National Government of the Netherlands, 2015b). A second example is the requirement of those receiving unemployment benefits in some municipalities to perform a "compensatory act" within their individual abilities in the Participation Act (National Government of the Netherlands, 2015a). In the relatively short period of time since its legal introduction, this has introduced strategic uncertainties with regards to accountability and liability, but it has also created room for experimentation and innovation.

Following recent decentralizations in long-term and social care with specific policy goals for prevention in the Health Insurance Act (2006), the revised Social Support Act (2015), the Youth Act (2015) and the Long Term Care Act (2015), municipalities now voice a *call for prevention in the local development* of integrated and capacitating neighbourhood service teams. Public health services, however, for a number of reasons seem to participate only to a limited extent. As opposed to these decentralizations, municipal public health services in the past thirty years have merged from 65 (1985) to 25 regional services against 390 municipalities (1 January 2017) so as to match the regional emergency preparedness teams. Community-based health promotion in the past ten years, moreover, was under heavy retrenchment, which leaves very limited means and support for neighbourhood team participation (Koornstra

& Stom, 2016). As a consequence, with some exceptions, public health services are still not well integrated into the local networks for care services and social support (Andersson Elffers Felix, 2013).

10.2.4 Public health challenges

Public health problems have posed new challenges to government and public health services in the Netherlands in the past ten years. With regard to vaccination policies and cancer screenings, for instance, government and services are faced with *declining trust in expert judgement* among citizens groups in the population who articulate and mobilize collective suspicion of health risks on social media (Wallenburg & Bal, 2008; Rondy et al., 2010). On the other hand there is a growing recognition in society of the need for *collective action* on public health, for instance on tackling the root causes of behaviour-related diseases and health conditions as a shared responsibility across the state, the market, the family and (organized) CSOs (Hendriks et al., 2013; Mackenbach, 2016). In the past ten years many citizen, community and commercial initiatives have been initiated, focusing on weight loss, physical activity, lifestyle coaching, etc. Although this exemplifies public awareness of the social determinants of lifestyle-related health problems, it has also led to fragmentation, inefficiency and a lack of transparency on the societal impact of public health-related initiatives (Tweede Kamer der Staten-Generaal, 2014).

10.2.5 A political opportunity

An opportunity for collective action on health presented itself when Parliament in 2012 asked the Ministry of Health to develop a National Prevention Plan (Tweede Kamer der Staten-Generaal, 2012). The Minister and State Secretary agreed and, in consultation with a broad representation of interests, developed the National Prevention Programme "All about Health…" (Ministery of Health, Welfare and Sport et al., 2013). It consists of (a) existing legal regulations; (b) a number of government-led health programmes, such as Healthy School, Youth on a Healthy Weight (JOGG), and Healthy in the City (GezondIn); and (c) a platform of pledges called "All about Health…". Below we will first describe the generic framework of the NPP: the platform of pledges and their emerging networks. We then describe the activities, processes and strategies, and the conditions for CSOs as emerging from the early "All about Health…" experiences.

10.3 "All about Health…" 2014–2016 and the role of civil society

In response to the challenges described above, the Dutch National Prevention Programme "All about Health…" (2014–2016) was initiated in an attempt to integrate public and private health initiatives. It was thought that fostering domain-crossing activities and knowledge exchange would increase the reach and impact of health promotion initiatives. We first describe the general framework, followed by observations on the actual practices developed in the pledges locally and in relation to the national Programme Office, the Ministry of Health, and other Ministries involved.

10.3.1 The "All about Health…" general framework

The general framework consists of ambitions, instruments, infrastructure and independent monitoring informing democratic accountability and programme improvement.

Long-term ambitions and settings

The "All about Health…" initiative aims to create a social "health movement" among equal participants in society, business, communities and governments at multiple levels with long-term health goals. By 2030 it aims to reduce chronic diseases by reversing the trends in six public policy priorities (smoking, alcohol abuse, diabetes, obesity, depression and physical exercise) (Ministry of Health, Welfare and Sport, 2011) and bringing the growing health disparities to a halt. The programme is categorized into four settings – school, work, living neighbourhood and health care – and separate attention is paid to health protection (Tweede Kamer der Staten-Generaal, 2013).

Partner pledges as a quasi-social contract

Partner commitment to the programme manifests itself in a pledge: "a public statement by which an organization expresses commitment and an active contribution to the realization of the NPP-Health goals by conducting specific focused activities" (www.allesisgezondheid.nl). In 2013 the programme was positioned explicitly as a joint initiative of six Ministries (Health, Welfare and Sport; Education and Cultural Affairs; Internal Affairs; Infrastructure and Environment; Social Affairs and Employment; and Economic Affairs). The government takes a non-hierarchical role and partners are primarily responsible: "It will be the art of being mutually inspiring and keeping each other focused and committed, making visible results and learning from experience without ending up in a stifling bureaucracy. This means there will be no single project organization with central decision-making and monitoring" (Tweede Kamer der Staten-Generaal, 2013, p. 16). Low entrance and limited requirements for participation are maintained so that partners, within the general health ambitions, can develop their own goals and activities even when these are sometimes perceived to be at a distance from being health-relevant, such as low literacy.

Infrastructure

A small facilitative Programme Office is funded by the coordinating Ministry of Health, populated by part-time, non-governmental account managers in the respective domains, and situated at a distance from the government seat in The Hague. The Office consists of two MoH-appointed officers and six temporary part-time *account managers* for the four domains (health protection being part of all domains). Other arrangements include a *partner platform* of representatives aimed at sharing experience with and advising the Programme Office, a number of *celebrity ambassadors* in sports, architecture (healthy urbanism), and social entrepreneurship. There are *regular meetings* and an *annual conference* presenting the pledges and their progress. The marketing and communication strategy consists of *social media*[4] making publicly visible the contributions of partners and offering opportunities for networking.

Independent monitoring and evaluation

Responsibilities for achieving the goals of the pledges are kept decentral, asking partners to be transparent about progress in an online survey once a year. Partners are asked to account for their activities among themselves in a dynamic and horizontal review: "Each partner is responsible for the activities and results in their own domain, can be questioned by other partners, and will account for their actions in public" (Tweede Kamer der Staten-Generaal, 2013, p. 16). The Dutch Organization of Health Research and Innovation (ZonMw) has set up three different and independent monitoring trajectories. There was a small-scale quantitative monitoring trajectory focusing mainly on process indicators (numbers of pledges, partners, activities, etc.); a qualitative governance-monitoring trajectory (of which this paper is a product); and an evaluation trajectory of implementation and health outcomes in nine single pledges.

---

4 http://www.allesisgezondheid.nl/; https://www.facebook.com/allesisgezondheid; https://twitter.com/AlGezondheid; https://www.linkedin.com/company/alles-is-gezondheid; https://www.youtube.com/user/allesisgezondheid; http://www.socialmarktplaats.net/.

10.3.2 Research methods

Since the programme is a relatively new phenomenon and had only recently started before our study took off, we decided to conduct a formative, action-oriented process evaluation. We first of all conducted an international scoping of literature about similar programmes (the Quebec "Investir pour l'avenir" programme and the UK Public Health Responsibility Deal programme), and a quick scan of similar Dutch programmes and evaluations (the economic Green Deals programme and the Corporate Social Responsibility Foundation)[5]. We then engaged in qualitative monitoring, consisting of (a) national level participant observations of Programme Office meetings, "All about Health…" events, and discussion with the Ministry of Health; and (b) a multiple case study design of six pledge partner networks selected to represent as much diversity in the "All about Health…" programme as possible. We additionally set up a digital marketing analysis of the five social media channels used in "All about Health…"; and in one of the cases conducted a responsive future scenario exploration with local partners. Finally, we provided feedback into the programme by regularly sharing our preliminary findings with programme officials. The results in this chapter are derived primarily from the literature scan and the case studies, and have been cross-checked with programme officials.

10.3.3 Results

Which activities do CSO partners of the 'All about Health…' programme contribute?

After three years the "All about Health…" programme has generated 309 pledges from 1825 partners in society[6] (see Fig. 10.1).

Strictly speaking, not all the "All about Health…" partners are CSOs. We roughly estimated that about half the partners are CSOs (mostly voluntary, not-for-profit organizations such as foundations, networks and alliances, and citizen initiatives, and a smaller proportion of private organizations with a public task and no profit-sharing, including care providers and insurers, educational and cultural organizations). About a third of the partners are *commercial* partners (individual entrepreneurs, small and large businesses). Finally, about 10% are *public* organizations, such as municipalities, government agencies and public health services. The juridical status of the remaining 5% is unknown to us. Some of the pledges formalize activities that have been going on for a long time, while other activities result from partner commitment in the "All about Health…" pledge.

---

5 www.quebecenforme.org; https://responsibilitydeal.dh.gov.uk/; www.greendeals.nl; www.mvonederland.nl .
6 www.allesisgezondheid.nl (in Dutch only).

Fig. 10.1 *Total amount of pledges and development over time, 2014–2016*

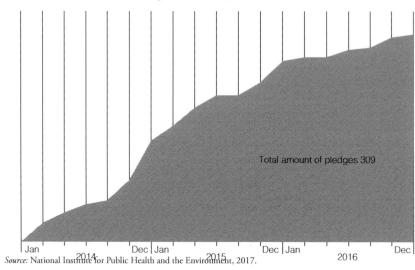

Source: National Institute for Public Health and the Environment, 2017.

The annual "All about Health…" Monitoring and Progress Report shows that around two-thirds of the pledges focus on promoting general lifestyle and behaviour, including sports and physical activity (see Fig. 10.2).

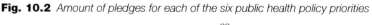

Fig. 10.2 *Amount of pledges for each of the six public health policy priorities*

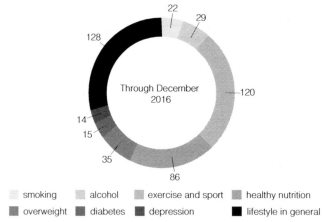

Source: National Institute for Public Health and the Environment, 2017.

Mental health and smoking are relatively underserved in the pledges but these are addressed in other activities outside the pledges. In 2015 partners reported that 20% of single pledges reached fewer than 100 people, 27% reached 100–1000 people, 27% reached 1000–10 000 people and another 20% more than 10 000 people. About 70% of partners actively work together with other domains, and this percentage is increasing (see Fig. 10.3).[7]

7 http://www.allesisgezondheid.nl/monitoring (in Dutch only).

Fig. 10.3 *Share of pledge partners actively working together with other domains*

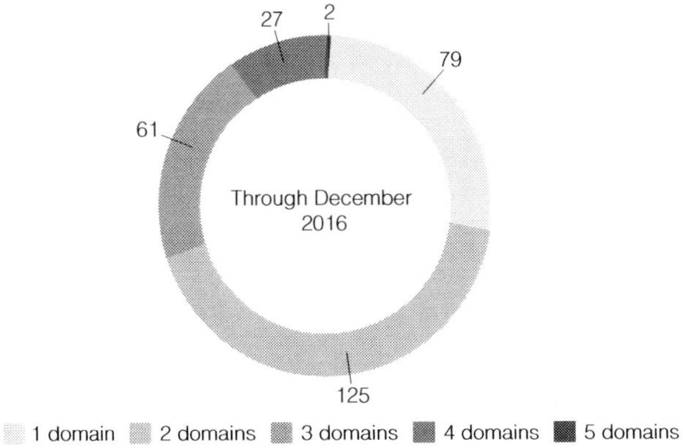

Through December 2016

27 2

79

61

125

1 domain 2 domains 3 domains 4 domains 5 domains

Source: National Institute for Public Health and the Environment, 2017.

In Chapter 2 of this book the matrix of CSOs distinguished between nine types of activity and roles CSOs may be involved with. In the "All about Health…" programme, we encounter examples of all of these nine types. First of all, *organizing services and events for members and the public* is the most prominent type of activity among all pledge partners. As an example, the Care Innovation Centre West-Brabant[8] organizes meetings and events for the elderly and other interested groups in their "House of Tomorrow" based in a school for vocational training, showcasing care innovations, offering free advice, and educating vocational health care students on health innovations and patient/consumer demands.

The Care Innovation Centre (CIC) is also exemplary of *being a key to industrial relations with the health sector*: the CIC made it its core business to engage industrial partners from the health innovation and design industry and link them up with consumer groups such as local associations for the elderly. In order to make this connection acceptable and effective, providing advice rather than selling products turned out to be crucial. The CIC literally fills the void between innovators and potential user groups, making possible user feedback and product improvement. The organizations in between, the health care providers, are also actively engaged in the network.

Thirdly, *helping consensus building* in all pledges is centred around creating awareness of health, disease prevention and the role and interest of non-health actors and organizations in and beyond the pledge. In the case of Deltion, a large school for broad vocational training with 15 000 students and about 1200 staff, the Sports education team took the initiative to introduce a

---

8 http://www.cic-westbrabant.nl/ (in Dutch only).

Vitality programme for students and staff. The Board has embraced this, and now all students undergo vitality tests and a healthy lifestyle education. The staff has access to a Vitality coach and participate in regular events. The Logistics educational department (for truck drivers, car mechanics, etc.) is now experimenting with an educational module on Vitality and sustainable labour participation, thereby also going into dialogue about this topic with businesses offering student internships.

The Sports team thus has also effectively built consensus and *contributed to Deltion's organizational policy development*: the Vitality ambition is part of the organizational mission statement that is displayed on banners throughout the school. Additionally, the school *acts as a self-regulator* with a large red carpet outside the entrance to the school, displaying the statement "smoke-free zone" (Fig. 10.4).

Fig. 10.4 *Deltion self-regulatory red carpet "smoke free zone"*

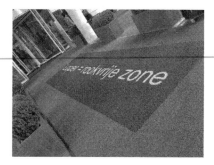

Source: M. Bekker.

In another pledge network, on implementing the concept of "Positive Health"[9] as an organizing principle of integrated primary and social care, general practitioners managed to negotiate contractual funding with care insurers for the coordination of this social (= organizational) innovation. This could be a first step towards organizational, insurance and municipal policies and contracts for integrated primary and social care.

Other activities of pledge partners include *providing evidence*: some pledges are centred around investing time and funding into research, or research is a by-product making the implementation of the pledge more transparent. For example, in a pledge from Heineken and the Sports Federation NOC-NSF about the prevention of alcohol abuse in sports canteens, Heineken organized the "Stay Clear" campaign. Heineken funded research into the impact of a peer youth visitor (aged around 18) in two subsequent "mystery visits" engaging in

---

9 Based on six stakeholder group consultations (doctors, nurses, patients, policy-makers, scientists and health care insurers), health was suggested to be redefined as the ability to adapt and self-manage in light of social, physical and emotional life challenges, such as disease, divorce or unemployment (Huber et al., 2011).

conversations with bar-tenders, providing information, education and feedback on alcohol abuse. Heineken also made available "Stay Clear" banners for sports canteens and initiated a contest for the best "Stay Clear" canteen. Based on the results, Heineken and NOC-NSF decided to continue their commitment and strengthen their intervention so as to improve impact.

In the long-standing collaboration between Heineken and the Sports Federation NOC-NSF, the latter also acts a *watch dog*, or rather as a *"moral counsellor"* pushing the former to be more ambitious, to take longer-term actions and to develop stronger interventions in social responsibility. This commercial and CSO partnership could be a first step towards a more fundamental balancing of public health values and commercial interests. For Heineken, as a multinational corporation, this is a relatively small activity, yet without it NOC-NSF would not be able to get this intervention funded and organized.

The Heineken "Stay Clear" banner for sports canteens: "Our club is clear: no alcohol under 18. Older than 18? Enjoy responsibly. When in doubt we will ask to show your ID. Bar tenders rule."

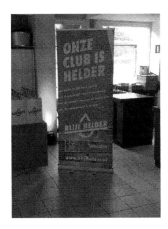

Source: T. Bosch.

Some of the pledge partners also engage in *exercising advocacy*; for instance, under the "flag" of "All about Health…" an alliance was forged around the problem of illiteracy. About 50 organizations joined the alliance to link up knowledge, resources and ambitions. The national Programme Office organized events around this theme and was also involved in regional or local pledge network activities raising awareness of illiteracy and its impact on health (and health disparities). One observed impact was an elected municipal Alderwoman taking up this topic as a priority in the municipal Health Policy memorandum.

Finally, most of the CSOs and other partners in the "All about Health…" programme offer *committed people, flexible working routines, and responsive service delivery.* At this early stage, dialogue and collaboration are centred mostly within the single pledge partner networks. Feedback between pledges, and with the Programme Office and the national government, is still occasional rather than structural and systematic. We elaborate on this in the next section.

How do governments and CSOs develop dialogue and collaboration in practice?

Partners' motivations to participate in "All about Health…" range from sharing a common challenge such as underperforming students or staff with risky lifestyles to sharing a good idea or innovative solution for integrating primary and social care, to maintaining good relationships with the Ministry of Health in order to be in a better position to avoid or co-develop regulations.

Most of the partner organizations invest many working hours. Other sources are made available through sharing knowledge and experience, and providing access to new partners and targeted groups by linking up different networks across domains. The level of commitment in such people is exceptionally high, as expressed in devoted private hours and compared to regular organizational or business activities. The coordinators are able to be "agile" and responsive to changing circumstances, as our process tracing has showed.

The pledges that were investigated in-depth all show an organic and pragmatic development of targeted activities, often in direct contact with the relevant risk or user groups. In order to keep the energy going, partners undertake action rather than build consensus and detailed project plans as these are (too) time-consuming. Partners actively reflect and learn from these experiences and adapt their strategy or approach. As a result, pledges' activities and networks address context-appropriate and thus very different topics and issues in many different ways with many different partners, and their networks develop at a different pace. Diversity in this programme is a powerful resource.

We observe that a small number of the pledges are conducted by a single partner and there is hardly any network development. A bigger proportion of the pledges display features of *explorative collaborations*. At this early stage partners build relationships and explore common ground for a general health ambition and more concrete goals that serve (or at least do not harm) the various interests. At this "goal-seeking" stage partners do not yet depend on each other and the stakes are relatively low. There are no obligations (yet) towards one another. This enables a growth of trust, intrinsic commitment and coherence. The explorative collaborations in some of the pledge networks thus advance to shared objectives, conditions and terms of engagement, such as self-monitoring and evaluation. Such *"entrepreneurial" collaborations* no longer need external incentives to keep things going and manifest a degree of "self-organization" (Kaats & Opheij, 2012; Bekker et al., 2016a).

While some partners conduct formal research, others engage with "reflexive dialogues and monitoring". Adapting and improving goals, strategies, perceptions and working routines, making them more appropriate and responsive, generate legitimacy and create room for social innovation of organizational structures, procedures, and rules. There is a call for scaling-up of good practices but there is hardly any evidence of this actually occurring. Because of context-appropriateness, good practices are not easily transferable to other settings. Another explanation is the lack of felt ownership in other settings. For each setting, combining elements of different good practices matching local utility, acceptance and feasibility seems more appropriate.

Pledge partners feel that the added benefits of the "pledge" as a coordinating instrument include the incentive to actually undertake action; the access it provides to new partners and the opportunities for new partnerships; the public stage for their ambitions and impacts in "All about Health…" social media posts; and the legitimacy that goes with participating in a national level platform in which various Ministries are involved. The latter in particular has helped partners to mobilize commitment from influential parties such as large municipalities or care insurers. At the same time there are also partners who expect more value in return for their investments.

Which conditions emerge enhancing the work of CSOs in "All about Health…"?

During the course of the first three years of "All about Health…" it became clear that a distinction drawn between the governmental programmes, municipal health policies and their implementation networks on the one hand and the "All about Health…" movement and pledges on the other hand, would clarify the different roles, responsibilities and accountabilities involved. In the policy implementation networks, the government takes a central top-down role in setting priorities and terms of implementation, such as supervision and control, but the role of government in the "All about Health…" networks is far more facilitative to CSO needs (Bekker et al., 2016a). External requirements, such as SMART-formulated objectives and quantitative monitoring, scaling-up and organizational consolidation of good practices, should be trimmed down to become realistic, appropriate and enabling conditions rather than disqualifiers that might paralyse practice.

In addition to facilitating the partners, "All about Health…" programme support (now the Programme Office) has several important functions (Bekker et al., 2016b):

- brokering cross-domain connections;
- organizing systematic on- and offline knowledge sharing and exchange;

- incentivizing new pledges and partners as well as strengthening the ambition in current pledges (while also accepting pledge closure when the pledge is fulfilled and partners no longer feel committed); and

- systematically collecting partner feedback and detecting signals about contradictory regulations or bureaucratic obstacles, as well as feeding back on follow up and actions taken.

Trust and reciprocity are crucial conditions. The pledge partners expect the government to be actively interested in their activities and achievements. They also want government to take a consistent position in this social health movement without constraining partners or judging whether their achievements are in line with government priorities or not. Most of the activities, if not all of them, contribute to the determinants of health. A low entrance for newcomers as diverse as possible remains important so as to keep the flow of innovative domain-crossing ideas going.

Democratic accountability remains important since network initiatives might, in the end, only serve their own partners' interests while the public issues and challenges of external groups remain unsolved. Transparent progress deliberation and horizontal, forward-looking accountability among equal partners secures ownership that is more conducive to adaptation and improvement (Sabel, 1993). The direct participation of citizens can help improve democratic legitimacy. Moreover, citizens are co-producers, not passive recipients of health, and so may well improve implementation and impact.

Programme monitoring and evaluation (Bryden et al., 2013) is also important as a touchstone for reflection, contextualization, comparison, and accountability. Additionally, elected politicians and representatives at the municipal, provincial and national level could be more actively invited to take part in reflexive work visits and dialogue tables with street level workers and risk or user groups. Learning about the many small steps towards impact and change might help to develop appropriate procedures and requirements for democratic accountability.

Finally, based on comparative research into similar programmes in other policy sectors and in Quebec and the UK, it generally takes at least five to ten years before such a "Whole of Society" programme produces irreversible conditions: having CSOs develop trusting and solid partnerships; developing a public attitude for domain-crossing actions; and establishing regulatory and other institutional conditions for a working routine that enables being and remaining responsive and conducive to social innovation (Dubé et al., 2014; Addy et al., 2014; Petticrew et al., 2013). Small successes count because they induce trust and continuity. Early experiences with "All about Health…" confirm that time, trust and reciprocity remain important conditions for bottom-up governance by CSOs, fostering innovation and change, towards a higher reach and impact on health (Bekker et al., 2016b).

10.4 Conclusion: from government to health governance

In this chapter we investigated the background, trends and early stage innovations in the relationship between CSOs, the market and the state in the Netherlands. We illustrated this with the recent programme "All about Health…" which created a platform of collaborative public, private and CSO initiatives for health.

The analysis of the first three years of "All about Health…" seems to provide an early backing of the hypothesis in this book about the potential of civil society organizations contributing to public health. In Chapter 1 of this book it was expected that "Civil society organizations (CSOs) tackle a large variety of diverse health issues and represent the interest of different constituencies including citizens, patients and stakeholders. They could offer committed people, flexibility, and responsiveness in service delivery that public sector and private sector organizations alike fail to muster. They could also mediate problematic policies; bring expertise, ideas, and diverse perspectives. Finally they would be seen to be more credible. Government would have to cope with more criticism and an element of unpredictability that comes with commitment and flexibility." Further details on how CSOs operate would, however, be dependent on the context of state-society relationships and were therefore not prescribed.

In the Netherlands state-society relationships consisted for a long time of corporatist organizations representing majority and minority interests in a consensual style of public policy-making. This corporatist tradition has eroded in favour of evidence-based policy-making with new or revised institutions at the policy-making table. The dominant public issue for decades had been reforming the health care system towards a regulated competition model. Disease prevention has been decoupled from health care for a long time and locked into the public sector, with little support from societal interests and a strong role for science-based public health institutes. In the past decade, however, challenges have evolved around *declining trust in public health expert judgement* and public recognition of the need for *collective action* on health problems. Health is rapidly becoming marketed, contributing to community awareness and demand, as well as to a fragmented health field. Recent government incentives are trying to introduce new forms of collective action among the state, the market and the community for health and other welfare issues. Experiments with a facilitative rather than controlling government provide early experience of opportunities and pitfalls.

The "All about Health…" programme, aiming to create a social health movement with CSO pledges to promote health and reduce health inequalities, is an early example of a "Whole of Society" approach. This approach indicates a shift from government to governance, attempting to reconcile state, market and society, economic and health interests, and public and private organizations. In so doing it is also seeking a reconciliation of ideas, interests and institutions. Its partners consist of CSOs, commercial businesses and public institutions working together in explorative cross-domain networks with an adaptive attitude in organic and pragmatic processes of learning by doing.

We have illustrated how the "All about Health…" partners provided evidence, contributed to policy development, exercised advocacy, helped consensus building, acted as watch dogs, provided services to members and to the public, acted as self-regulators and were key in industrial relations in the health sector. They have offered committed people, flexibility, and responsiveness in service delivery. They mostly did so in close collaborative relationships across different domains developing from explorative towards entrepreneurial networks. Nevertheless, in the long run these core features of early networks in the "All about Health…" programme are vulnerable. Legitimizing new working routines across the partners and domains could be one way of consolidating the rewards, values and impacts of the "All about Health…" pledge activities.

A final condition to making civil society work for health is to have research scientists who are capable of conducting independent, yet action-oriented and contextualized evaluations based on qualitative and responsive research methods in order to reconstruct its meaning across different settings. Based, among other sources, on this research, on 4 November 2016 the Ministry of Health sent a letter to Parliament deciding on a five-year extension of "All about Health…" (Ministry of Health, Welfare and Sport, 2016) . While it is still too early to present the "All about Health…" programme as a successful governance innovation, it certainly is a courageous, challenging and promising addition to the traditional systems, patterns and routines of public health policy and practice.

Acknowledgements

We would like to express our gratitude and indebtedness to, first of all, Inge Lecluijze, Tjisse Bosch and Marieke Verhorst, who collected the data in five of the six case studies and participated in the analysis. Many thanks to Cathy Rompelberg and Matthijs van den Berg for providing us with the latest figures on the quantitative progress indicators. We thank Tom van der Grinten, Robin Bremekamp and Hans van Oers for their useful advice on our study. We finally thank Jack Hutten, Henk Soorsma, Sonja Bleulandt and Victor Stöcker for facilitating the implementation of this study.

References

Addy NA et al. (2014). Whole-of-Society Approach for Public Health Policymaking: A Case Study of Polycentric Governance from Quebec, Canada. *Ann N Y Acad Sci.*, 1331: 216–229.

Andersson Elffers Felix (2013). Borging van de Publieke Gezondheid En de Positie van de GGD [Public Health and GGD Position]. Utrecht, Andersson Elffers Felix (https://repub.eur.nl/pub/10813, last accessed 28 January 2017).

Bekker M, Putters K (2003). Sturing van Lokaal Gezondheidsbeleid: De Verknoping van Gescheiden Netwerken [Governance of local health policy: the cross linking of separate networks]. In Bekkers V et al. eds., *Handboek Voor de Sociale Sector*, 9–10 (https://repub.eur.nl/pub/10813, last accessed 27 January 2017).

Bekker M et al. (2010). Linking Research and Policy in Dutch Healthcare: Infrastructure, Innovations and Impacts. *Evidence & Policy: A Journal of Research, Debate and Practice*, 6(2):237–253. doi:10.1332/174426410X502464.

Bekker M. et al. (2016a). Healthy Networks in the National Prevention Program 'All about Health...' (Gezonde Netwerken in Het Nationaal Programma Preventie 'Alles Is Gezondheid...'). *Dutch J Health Sc/T Gezondheidswetenschappen*, 94(4):128–130.

Bekker M et al. (2016b). Appendix to Letter of the MoH to Parliament No. 32793-245: Preliminary Findings of the University of Maastricht Study into the "All about Health..." Programme. The Hague, National Government of the Netherlands (https://www.rijksoverheid.nl/documenten/rapporten/2016/11/03/voorlopige-hoofdpunten-studie-gezondheid-door-sturing-borging-en-verantwoording-in-het-nationaal-programma-preventie-alles-is-gezondheid, last accessed 27 January 2017).

Brandsen T, Pape U (2015). The Netherlands: The Paradox of Government–Nonprofit Partnerships. *VOLUNTAS: International Journal of Voluntary and Nonprofit Organizations*, 26(6):2267–2282. doi:10.1007/s11266-015-9646-3.

Bryden A et al. (2013). Voluntary Agreements between Government and Business – a Scoping Review of the Literature with Specific Reference to the Public Health Responsibility Deal. *Health Policy*, 110(2–3):186–197.

Carroll AB (1991). The Pyramid of Corporate Social Responsibility: Toward the Moral Management of Organizational Stakeholders. *Business Horizons*, 34(4):39–48. doi:10.1016/0007-6813(91)90005-G.

Dubé L et al. (2014). From Policy Coherence to 21st Century Convergence: A Whole-of-Society Paradigm of Human and Economic Development. *Ann N Y Acad Sci.*, 1331:201–215.

Helderman JK (2007). Bringing the Market Back In? Institutional Complementarity and Hierarchy in Dutch Housing and Health Care [PhD thesis]. Rotterdam, Erasmus Universiteit Rotterdam.

Helderman JK, Bevan G, France G (2012). The Rise of the Regulatory State in Health Care. A Comparative analysis of Britain, the Netherlands and Italy. *Health Economics, Policy and Law*, 7(1):103–124.

Helderman JK et al. (2005). Market-oriented health care reforms and policy learning in the Netherlands. *Journal of Health Politics, Policy and Law*, 30(1/2):189–209.

Hemerijck AC (1992). The historical contingencies of Dutch corporatism. PhD dissertation, Oxford, Oxford, University (Balliol College).

Hendriks A et al. (2013). Towards Health in All Policies for Childhood Obesity Prevention. *Journal of Obesity*, 2013 (ID 632540):12.

Huber M et al. (2011). How Should We Define Health? *BMJ (Clinical Research Ed.)*, 343:d4163. doi:10.1136/bmj.d4163.

Jong P, van den Brink M (2013). Between Tradition and Innovation: Developing Flood Risk Management Plans in the Netherlands. *Journal of Flood Risk Management*, 10:155–163. doi:10.1111/jfr3.12070.

Kaats E, Opheij W (2012). *Leren Samenwerken Tussen organisaties. Samen Bouwen Aan Allianties, Netwerken, Ketens En Partnerships [Learning to collaborate between organizations – Alliances – networks – chains – partnerships]*. Deventer: Kluwer.

Koornstra A, Stom C (2016). Publieke Gezondheid Borgen. Een Eerste Inzicht in de Staat van GGD'en *[Public Health. A first insight into the state of local health authorities]*. Utrecht (https://www.ggdghorkennisnet.nl/thema/publieke-gezondheid-borgen/nieuws/6173-publieke-gezondheid-borgen-kansen-voor-versterking, last accessed 27 January 2017).

Mackenbach JP (2003). Sociale geneeskunde en 'public health': historische kanttekeningen bij de Nederlandse situatie [Social medicine and 'public health': historic question marks to the Dutch situation]. *Dutch Journal of Health Sciences*, 91(3):450–458.

Mackenbach JD (2016). Exploring Obesogenic Environments: The Role of Environmental Factors for Obesity-Related Behaviours and Obesity. Amsterdam, PhD, Vrije Universiteit Amsterdam. http://dare.ubvu.vu.nl/handle/1871/54633, last accessed 27 January 2017.

Ministry of Economic Affairs, Agriculture & Innovation (2012). Voortgangsrapportage Green Deals 2012 [Progress Report Green Deal 2012]. The Hague, Ministry of Economic Affairs, Agriculture & Innovation, letter from the Minister.

Ministry of Health, Welfare and Sport (2011). Health close to the people. Policy document The Hague, Ministry of Health, Welfare and Sport.

Ministry of Health, Welfare and Sport et al. (2013). *Het Nationale Preventie Programma "Alles Is Gezondheid" 2014–2016* ["All about Health …" The National Prevention Programme 2014–2016]. *Kamerstuk 2013D40425.* The Hague, Tweede Kamer der Staten-Generaal.

Ministry of Health, Welfare and Sport (2016). Letter from the MoH to Parliament, 3 November 2016, on the Extension of the National Prevention Programme 'All about Health...'. The Hague: Tweede Kamer der Staten-Generaal (https://www.rijksoverheid.nl/documenten/kamerstukken/2016/11/03/kamerbrief-over-vervolg-nationaal-programma-preventie-en-alles-is-gezondheid, last accessed 27 January 2017).

MVO Nederland (2013). Geïntegreerd Jaarverslag 2012 [Integrated Annual Report 2012]. Utrecht, MVO Nederland.

National Government of the Netherlands (2013). Troonrede 2013 [Speech from the Throne 2013] (https://www.rijksoverheid.nl/documenten/toespraken/2013/09/17/troonrede-2013, last accessed 28 January 2017).

National Government of the Netherlands (2015a). *Participation Act.* Amsterdam, the National Government of the Netherlands (http://wetten.overheid.nl/BWBR0015703/2017-02-01, last accessed 28 January 2017).

National Government of the Netherlands (2015b). *Youth Act.* Amsterdam, the National Government of the Netherlands (http://wetten.overheid.nl/BWBR0034925/2016-08-01, last accessed 28 January 2017).

National Institute for Public Health and the Environment (2017). Voortgangsmonitoring [Progress Monitoring]. In National Institute for Public Health and the Environment (RIVM), *Drie Jaar "Alles Is Gezondheid...",* Amersfoort.

Petticrew M et al. (2013). The Public Health Responsibility Deal: How Should Such a Complex Public Health Policy Be Evaluated? *J Pub Health*, 35(4): 495–501.

Putters K, van Twist MJT (2007). Bijdragen Aan Beleid of Tegenspel Bieden? Modaliteiten Voor Een Vernieuwd Adviesstelsel *[Contributing to, or rethinking policy? Modalities for a revised Advisory Council system]*. *Tijdschr. Bestuurswetenschappen*, 61(2):11–19.

Rondy M et al. (2010). Determinants for HPV Vaccine Uptake in the Netherlands: A Multilevel Study. *Vaccine*, 28(9):2070–2075. doi:10.1016/j. vaccine.2009.12.042.

Sabel CF (1993). Learning by Monitoring. The Institutions of Economic Development. New York, Columbia University School of Law, Working paper 102.

Tweede Kamer der Staten Generaal (2012). *Motie van de Leden Dijkstra En Bruins Slot. 33400 XVI 69. Vergaderjaar 2012–2013 [Members motion Pia Dijkstra and Bruins Slot. Adoption of the budget of the Ministry of Health, Welfare and Sport (XVI) for the year 2013].* The Hague.

Tweede Kamer der Staten-Generaal (2013). Alles Is Gezondheid… Het Nationaal Programma Preventie 2014–2016. Kamerstuk 2013D40425. The Hague, Tweede Kamer der Staten-Generaal.

Tweede Kamer der Staten-Generaal (2014). Lijst van Vragen En Antwoorden Bij Het Nationaal Preventie Programma [List of questions and answers about the National Prevention Programme 2014–2016 – Preventive Health Policy]. Kamerstuk 2014D01858. The Hague.

van Mil et al. (2013). Externe Audit Green Deal Aanpak [External audit of the Green Deal approach]. The Hague, National Government of the Netherlands.

Wallenburg I, Bal RA (2008). Een nieuw vaccin in het Rijksvaccinatieprogramma? Kennisverzameling en besluitvorming in actie [A new vaccine in the National Vaccine Programme? Knowledge collection and decision-making in action.] The Hague, Rathenau Instituut.

Case study 7

From personal stories to policy action: a public campaign for improved obstetric care in Poland*

Erica Barbazza, Kerry Waddell

Out-dated care practices and sub-optimal standards of obstetric care in the early 1990s in Poland fuelled growing concern among women. Through informal exchanges, women found commonalities in their experiences, describing limited opportunities to discuss birthing preferences, such as determining birthing positions or making choices regarding treatment administered during labour, as well as a general absence of information on treatment and the rights of women.

In an effort to shed light on suboptimal obstetric services a group of motivated and concerned women partnered with the largest national daily newspaper, *Gazeta Wyborcza*. In doing so, they set out to turn shared experience into evidence and, in parallel, to ignite widespread public dialogue on this largely taboo topic. In 1994 the campaign was launched, inviting women to write to the newspaper about their childbirth experience. The public's response was overwhelming. In the first year over 2000 responses were received, but there were 50 000 responses in the following year.

From this, an understanding on the collective concern with current standards in obstetric services was established, and ultimately the foundation Childbirth with Dignity took shape. Set up by the campaign's organizers, the foundation aimed to advocate for changes on the issues brought forward by women and to empower them with information and support to express their needs and exercise their rights.

To accelerate political action for their cause, in 2006 the foundation released a ground-breaking report entitled Childbirth with Dignity is not a Privilege. The report highlighted key issues faced during childbirth, giving testimonials from over 26 000 women, as well as the views of health providers. In response to the report, the Ministry of Health convened an expert working group in 2007 to develop new

---

* For further details, see: WHO Regional Office for Europe (2016). Lessons from transforming health services delivery: Compendium of initiatives in the WHO European Region. Copenhagen: WHO Regional Office for Europe. (http://www.euro.who.int/en/health-topics/Health-systems/health-service-delivery/publications/2016/lessons-from-transforming-health-services-delivery-compendium-of-initiatives-in-the-who-european-region-2016).

obstetric care standards and, after several years of deliberation, the first Perinatal and Postnatal Care Standards were published in 2011.

At present, the foundation works closely with providers to increase their awareness of new guidelines and a general understanding of women's needs through regular training. The foundation also publishes educational resources for women on their web site and hosts an online database of reviews on experiences at facilities across the country. Since this first started, testimonials indicate women's childbirth experiences have improved, along with the provision of obstetric services according to best-available evidence.

Conclusion

This case illustrates the power of the public's voice, the potential of evidence to build momentum for change and challenge social conventions, and the ability of a few passionate individuals to take on the status quo and, through an evolving process, establish a public structure to accelerate improvements in services.

Case study 8

**Harnessing the power of celebrity disability –
getting people to see you, not through you**

Natasa Maros, Melita Murko

MyRight – Empowers people with disabilities (http://www.myright.ba/home) is an umbrella organization within the disability movement which works at the request of 30 member organizations to strengthen the local partner organizations' ability to run effective advocacy work. Since 2009 it has been active in Bosnia and Herzegovina, where its mission is to bring together 65 disabled persons' associations (DPOs), build their capacity, and create a joint platform for public awareness-raising and advocacy.

In a transitional, post-war country like Bosnia and Herzegovina, people with disabilities are not high on the political agenda nor visible in the media. Because of this general lack of public and government interest, and in the context of its monitoring of the UN Convention on the Rights of Persons with Disabilities (CRPD) implementation, the association decided to build a new type of media campaign to show persons with disabilities in a different light.

The campaign is about inspiring disabled people and others to take their rights seriously and is called "PonosniNaSebe" ("Proud of ourselves"). It highlights individual examples of people living with – and not being defined by – disability, making contributions to culture, art, science, and their communities. Disabled people are portrayed as people with talents and achievements, and not just their disabilities, and with the same rights as everybody else.

High-profile individuals with disabilities told their stories in MyRight's campaign and one of the biggest successes for the campaign came when Stephen Hawking supported the initiative by sending a personal message: *"I have motor neurone disease which has paralysed me. If I can succeed, others can as well."*

This initiative had a great impact, triggering significant media attention and many "likes" and "shares" on social media. This resulted in more people with disabilities being invited into television studios to talk about the campaign, their lives, hopes and challenges, and their right to participate as equals in society.

The campaign eventually also drew political attention, with politicians recognizing the need for legal and policy change.